"If you are very fortunate on your healing journey, you will occasionally encounter a healer who is constantly expanding his or her knowledge, and constantly working on himself or herself to become a wiser and more compassionate human being. Jeanette Bronée is such a guide, counselor, and healer. Heartfelt, down-to-earth, and deeply committed, she has used her remarkable skills to bring thousands of people through the many stages of healing. Her new book, *Eat to Feel Full (and Nourish Yourself for Good)*, is the progeny of that same wisdom. Read this book, learn to eat wisely and well, and heal yourself for good."

— Tom Monte
Author, *The Complete Guide to Natural Healing*

ISBN: 978-0-9863180-0-9

Printed in the United States of America
Design by goodutopian
Cover photograph by Torkil Stavdal
Bowl by Clay by DF

10 9 8 7 6 5 4 3 2

First Edition

EAT TO FEEL FULL

and nourish yourself for good

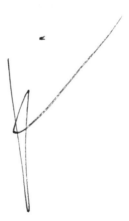

JEANETTE BRONÉE, CHHC

Founder, Path for Life

CONTENTS

INTRODUCTION:
HUMAN NATURE, FOOD AND YOU

Our Basic Human Design 16

The Nature of Hunger............................. 17

Appetite, Hunger & Self-Nourishment.......... 22

WHAT TO EAT:
KEYS TO MASTERING YOUR APPETITE

Vegetables: Food of the Earth........................ 29

Nature's Abundance 35

The Nurture of Green 36

Types of Leafy Greens 39

The Mighty Cruciferous:
Queen of the Veggies 43

Onions: Food & Medicine............................ 45

The Roots of Nurture................................ 46

Grains: The Daily Grain, Not the Daily Bread. 50

Wholegrain Facts at a Glance 58

Whole & Grainy Choices............................. 60

Protein: What, How & Why 63

Protein, Digestion & Appetite....................... 69

Dairy.. 70

The Skinny on Fats................................. 72

The Good, the Not-So-Good & the Ugly.......... 75
Fruit: The Sweet Nectar of Nature 84
Vitamins & Minerals.................................... 89
Health by Color 98
Superfoods for Mastering Appetite 104
Real Food for the Real You 117
The Balanced Meal: Putting It All Together ... 125
Hydration 128

HOW TO EAT:
FEELING MORE NOURISHED FROM YOUR FOOD
Good Eating 135
Mindful Eating 145
The Great Big Food Traps 146
Eating More or Less 154
Reading Labels 158
The Self-Nourishment Diet 163
The Food-Mind-Body Connection................... 163

COOKING BASICS
Brown Rice/Ancient Grains 169
Cooked Root Vegetables............................... 171
Roasted Cauliflower 172
Sautéed Red Cabbage 173
Sautéed Greens.. 174
Sautéed Onions & Leeks 175
Marinated Kale Salad 176

Lentil Salad 177
Cooked Beans 179
Tempeh 180
Whole Roasted Fish 181
Fish & Greens 182

SHOPPING LIST 187

AFTERWORD..197

ACKNOWLEDGMENTS 199

"We tend to judge our experience as good or bad and our hunger as emptiness or fullness. There is so much in between to notice and be mindful of. When we can slow down and pay attention to what's inside of us, we can have a fuller experience of who we are."

—Jeanette Bronée

EAT TO FEEL FULL

and nourish yourself for good

"Just like our predecessors, when we see and smell food we are triggered to take advantage of it."

INTRODUCTION

Human Nature, Food, and You

As you start reading this book, I am going to ask you first to pause, close your eyes, and say the word "food."

As you say it, notice what comes up for you. Notice how you feel in your body: There might be a sensation that rises in your stomach, throat, or chest. What does it feel like? You don't need to do anything about the feeling. This is how you'll start to get familiar with the way or ways the subject of food resonates for you. You may experience feelings of longing, fear, and anxiety, feelings of comfort and happiness, or a mixture. It's normal to have strong and even contradictory sensations about something so central to our lives. So what feelings come up for you when you think about food?

○

This book is a guide, full of information and tools that you can put to use immediately to change the way you eat. We'll cover WHAT to eat, WHEN and HOW. So why am I asking you to take stock of your feelings first? Each of us has a unique relationship to food; the way you relate to food is founded on your upbringing and your memories about the role of food in your childhood. For you to learn to eat in a satisfying way, it helps to be mindful of your *existing* relationship with food. This will help you decode the complicated mixed messages that tend to infuse our eating lives, so you can find the foods that truly nourish you.

Today, you eat a certain way based on choices you have or haven't made along the way, combined with a number of environmental and biographical factors that make up your food "heritage." Maybe you base your food choices mostly on convenience. Maybe you sense that you could be eating and feeling better, but you're uncertain what foods are best for you. Maybe you eat for pure pleasure or for the primordial need to satisfy hunger. Each of us is different.

This book will help you understand how to feel physically more satisfied from the food you eat. It won't prescribe a perfect diet, for a simple reason: There isn't one. "Eating better" will mean something different to each of us. You, and only you, will know when you are eating what's best *for you.* You'll know by your answers to these questions:

- Do you feel more satisfied from your food?

- Do you feel more energy after eating?

- Do you feel calmer, more centered and focused after a meal?

- Do you feel healthier?

When looking inward for these answers, remember that satisfaction is more than just the way you feel physically after a meal. To fully understand your overall sense of satisfaction—and to access the sense of well-being that comes with feeling satiated—you'll have to tap into your emotional world. Why? Because it's all too easy to confuse feelings of satisfaction or dissatisfaction about *food* with feelings of satisfaction and dissatisfaction about *life.* The clearer we can get on that distinction, the easier it is for us to take care of ourselves, and the healthier—and happier—we become.

The emotional aspects of eating are worthy of their own book. But this book is focused on the essential first step: FOOD KNOWLEDGE.

Food knowledge is more than just information; it's a way to understand how food affects you and to interpret those moments when you may think that, separate from true satiety, eating some particular food will *make you feel better*. It will teach you how to replace those unhelpful associations with real knowledge about how you can eat to feel full. And it will help you develop an appreciation of the art of eating.

Now, close your eyes again for a moment and check in with your body. Do you feel satisfied? Are you feeling a sense of emptiness inside? Are you hungry? Whatever you feel, just notice it, stay with it. It's time to learn how to relate to your own hunger.

OUR BASIC HUMAN DESIGN

Our bodies are fantastic machines. Like a dazzling network of information pathways, they are constantly communicating, interacting, and working for us. Think of a computer, of the wealth of information that can be stored in a tiny machine and the multitude of wonders it can do for us. Now think of this: *Your body is more amazing than any computer.*

Your body's information system doesn't only consist of the hunger signal we feel when considerable time has passed since our last meal. Each cell in your body—an estimated 50 to 100 trillion, depending on your age—is constantly working to maintain communication and balance. We don't sense this intense work but maybe if we did, we would trust this information and signaling system more. What we can do is learn how to understand our bodies better and choose how to feed them accordingly. When we do so from a self-nourishment perspective, the result is a feeling of deep satiety.

THE NATURE OF HUNGER

Human beings are built for survival. Our information system—a network of neurotransmitters within our bodies—was created to protect us, even if we don't always understand its inner workings.

Think about the dawn of human history. What were the most pressing daily concerns for our distant ancestors? Procuring food must have been near the top of the list, along with shelter, safety and procreation. Today, a top concern for most people is making money—which is how we meet our needs, including the still-essential need for food.

But while the methods we use to get food (buying it rather than hunting, gathering, or growing it) have changed—along with the levels of supply and demand in much of the world—our bodies have retained their ancient habits. Just like our predecessors, when we see and smell food we are triggered to take advantage of it. This is one reason we want to eat pretty much any time we walk by that kebab stand on the corner, even if we aren't hungry, even if we don't like kebabs. The indirect message encoded in our DNA is: "Take it! You don't know when there will be food again." Even if for many of us, going without access to food for an entire day or even a few hours is an implausibility, our survival instincts still respond in this primordial way. My grandmother always said, "You can't eat in advance." She was right, but our survivor instinct is, in a sense, telling us to do just that.

Another important neurotransmitter function is to check in with the stomach roughly every thirty minutes for signs of hunger. If you're under stress, it's easy to miss one or more of these periodic check-ins and not realize you're hungry until suddenly you're famished. If you are more present in your body (mindful), you'll notice a return signal saying "Yes," "Almost," or "Soon." The brain then "files" this information and checks in again half an hour later: Are you hungrier now? This cycle occurs in order to prepare us to find food well in advance of actually needing it. When this system of checking in evolved, procuring food was not so easy. These days, most of us just need to walk to the fridge or to the corner store. In effect, human evolution hasn't caught up to societal change; as a result, many of us react immediately to the earliest rumblings of hunger, and since food is plentiful and we can almost always get to it immediately, we eat too much, too fast—*before we are even truly hungry.*

◉

Here's the crucial thing to remember: The human body checks for signals of hunger *every thirty minutes.* The early signs are warning signs; they aren't saying "eat now" but, rather, "maybe it's time to think about what and where to eat next."

The benefit to listening to the early signs and interpreting them correctly is that if you do so, you can ensure that by the time you really *are* hungry—maybe an hour or so after the first warning signs—you've put yourself in a situation where you can access the foods you know are best for you to eat.

Another crucial aspect of this system is this: The difference between real hunger and the early warning signs is that the warning signs go away, then return with greater intensity after about thirty minutes.

So how can we respond to the small signals of early hunger without doing the obvious—eating mindlessly? Drinking water is a good immediate action, as it keeps the body hydrated (which is important anyway) while taking care of the first hunger pangs. But the most important thing to do is to train yourself to let the early hunger pangs trigger *mindful planning* instead of *immediate eating*. Instead of reaching for a snack, plan and prepare (or figure out where to get) a real, satisfying meal *in about an hour*.

This switch from eating to planning will help you be mindful about your choices, while preventing the panic-induced eating that occurs when real, overwhelming hunger strikes unexpectedly and we devour just about anything in sight.

◎

But how do we recognize hunger? And, more specifically, how can we tell the difference between real hunger and emotional hunger, which can trigger bouts of emotional eating?

We've all experienced the "artificial hunger" that can be caused by boredom, sadness, anger, and many other emotional states. We know from experience that eating can provide a momentary distraction from these unpleasant feelings. But we also know that no matter how hard we try, consciously or unconsciously, we can never satisfy emotion-based hunger by eating food—even healthy, wholesome food. Food alone cannot fill an emotional void.

Luckily, real hunger actually *feels physically different* than emotional hunger does—and you can learn how to recognize the difference.

If you are one of the countless many people who experience emotional hunger, the first step is to acknowledge it. There are resources available on the Path for Life website, including an online program specifically designed to help you understand and overcome habits related to emotional eating. Meanwhile this book, by teaching you the fundamentals about eating to feel full, can be the first step on your path toward healing.

In these pages, I focus on physical hunger and teach you a variety of techniques for mastering your appetite. You'll learn which food choices will keep you satisfied over a longer period of time, which means you will learn to master, and not be mastered by, your body's relationship to hunger.

APPETITE, HUNGER & SELF-NOURISHMENT

All hunger, whether physical or emotional, shows up as an *appetite for food*. Sometimes this becomes excessive, even overwhelming; other times, we have just a faint desire for something to munch on. *Physical hunger* is a sensation in the stomach, which includes pangs and sounds. A *craving* is felt differently—it's more like an idea in your mind of the thing that you suddenly crave—and it will usually last for only about ten minutes. On the scale of slight appetite to extreme hunger, we will always have a range of feelings. To master your appetite, you'll want to learn how *to recognize your personal point of satisfaction.* Once you become familiar with your own appetite, you will know how long you have from the very first signal until you should actually get some food. Reacting either too early or too late can lead to overeating.

It's always best to eat before your hunger becomes excessive. If it reaches that point, it can trigger the stress hormone cortisol, which will then cause you to react as if you're about to starve to death. The two hormones that normally tell you when you're hungry and full—gherlin and leptin—are suppressed when cortisol levels rise. The result is that if you've gotten too hungry, your appetite will feel limitless and you'll overeat as soon as you have the chance. This is pure biology—your body's survival instinct kicking in to save you from starvation. You can't change the biological mechanism, but fortunately you can learn to be mindful of it, and then it's much easier to avoid setting it off in the first place!

Our goal is to establish a balanced approach to eating, one that honors a healthy, natural relationship to hunger and satiety.

Recognizing your personal point of satisfaction means becoming aware of a number of different levels of hunger and knowing what to do when you reach each one—also, knowing which ones to avoid reaching altogether!

So before you move on to the next chapter, take a moment to think about how you feel in the following states:

> Slightly hungry
> Hungry
> No longer hungry
> Satisfied
> Full
> Stuffed

Now keep these states and your experience of them in mind as we move on to the core of this book: learning how to eat to feel full.

→ Train yourself to let early hunger pangs trigger mindful planning instead of immediate eating.

→ Remember that food alone cannot fill an emotional void.

"The higher the nutritional value of your food source, the more satisfied you feel."

WHAT TO EAT

Keys to Mastering Your Appetite

Eat whole, eat real, eat slowly, eat right, eat this and not that, eat sitting down, eat mindfully, eat with all your senses. Easier said than done, right? Let's take it one step at a time.

First: the issue of carbohydrates. Are all carbs bad? The answer to this is easy: No! In fact, *you cannot live without carbs.* The question I am going to answer here instead is: Which carbs are good for you and which carbs are best avoided? This may surprise you, but the first item on my good-carb list is: vegetables.

VEGETABLES: FOOD OF THE EARTH

Eat more vegetables. You've heard this before. You probably don't want to hear it again. But maybe some part of this instruction has been lost in transmission until now, so I'll ask you to listen to it one more time.

The official recommendation is 3-5 vegetable servings per day. I actually suggest 3-5 servings *twice* per day. That's because the highest levels of nutrients, vitamins, and minerals we can get from food are found in the plant and vegetable kingdom. The higher the nutritional value in your food source, the more satisfied you feel. Your body pays attention constantly; your intestinal tract continuously feeds your blood from what you eat. So what you eat governs much more than the feeling in your stomach; what you eat governs how you feel, how much energy you have—even how you think. And of course, it affects your overall health too.

All vegetables are not created equal. Studies have shown that most Americans believe they are eating a diet high in vegetables when they include iceberg lettuce, a slice of tomato, and a helping of potato chips in their evening meal. That is not the case! In fact, these are examples of vegetables that provide very low amounts of one of the most important elements of a satisfying meal: dietary fiber.

Fiber makes us feel full, and it also helps in cleansing the intestinal tract of waste, which in turn helps you to better absorb the nutrients in your food. Vegetables can be very high in fiber, but only when consumed in their whole state; many forms of food processing remove some or all of the fiber from the original food (think of what remains behind in the juicer after you've been served a green juice). Most processed bread products are also empty of the fiber that exists in the whole grains from which their main ingredient—usually flour—is derived.

Not only do vegetables—in their whole state with their fiber intact—help keep the intestines clean and healthy, they help us feel full and satisfied for longer after a meal, and they give us a lot of energy.

How does eating vegetables translate to more energy? That brings us back to good carbs, also known as *complex carbohydrates*.

Carbohydrates, whether simple or complex, are metabolized by our bodies and delivered into our bloodstreams as glucose. The problem arises when we eat simple carbohydrates, most commonly found in refined foods like sugar and many dairy products, and in vegetables and grains from which the fiber (and often the vitamins and minerals) has been removed in processing. These simple carbs are absorbed directly into the bloodstream with nothing to slow them down, which can wreak havoc on our energy levels. What sustains our energy for the long haul is complex carbohydrates. I will return to this in more detail in the chapter about grains, but the point to remember for now is that whole vegetables provide cleansing fiber and lasting energy via complex (good) carbohydrates.

Vegetables are also important for our hormones. The complex carbohydrates increase serotonin, which is the hormone that enhances mood and provides a sense of balanced well-being. So vegetables are your tool for feeling better on a daily basis and enhancing your general satisfaction. Mother was right: Eat your vegetables!

Many people believe that vegetables alone won't make them feel full—for that, they need their "meat and potatoes." To understand what's misleading about this reasoning, we just need to clarify *why* meat and potatoes seem more filling. A meal must contain fats and protein to be truly satisfying and to ward off hunger until the next meal. It's true that meat provides both fat and protein, but that's only part of the story. The fact is: *You can get your necessary fat and protein from plant-based foods too!*

Let's look at the difference. Meat does feel dense in the body, which gives it the impression of being substantial and satisfying. It also takes longer to break down (since it contains no cleansing fiber, meat can stick around in our digestive tracts for days). But we just said that foods that absorb too quickly—like simple carbohydrates—are not supportive for our energy levels, so wouldn't the slower pace of meat be a good thing? For some people it is, in small doses—and this is something you'll want to pay attention to as you get to know your appetite and satiety levels. But keep in mind that meat can go too far in the other direction, and if you eat a meal based almost entirely in meat and fat, you'll probably find that your energy drops while your body slows down to handle it.

Vegetables and plant fats, on the other hand, provide you with more directly usable energy since there isn't any conversion needed before the body is able to absorb the amino acids and vitamins; meat, by contrast, needs to be broken down into usable amino acids before its energy becomes available to the body. This also produces more waste than with plant-based protein.

There's a reason I recommend packing each meal with dense, fiber-rich vegetables. After a meal abundant with them, you will feel energized—instead of needing a siesta.

If you need any more convincing, here's what vegetables have going for them:

- Vegetables burn faster, meaning they are metabolized into energy (calories) more quickly and efficiently than are meat and fat. Our muscles run on complex carbohydrates, and even our brain needs carbohydrates for thinking. The fiber in vegetables and the fact that they provide complex (rather than simple) carbohydrates means that the release of energy is more immediate than with meat but slower and more lasting than with refined foods. Vegetables are the perfect fuel.

- Vegetables are generally low in calories and high in nutritional value. So, you can eat more of them if you need to without adding a lot of calories.

- Most vegetables are digested within three to four hours, which is the perfect interval between meals (more to come on that topic later on).

NATURE'S ABUNDANCE

If you go to a farmers' market, you might notice the abundance of the vegetable kingdom. The supermarket will also show you a large selection, but it's at the farmers' market that you'll find only the vegetables that are being harvested at that moment: *seasonal vegetables*. Before refrigeration and long-distance food distribution, we only had access to what was in season; we would pickle these seasonal vegetables to preserve them for later use. With the growing modernization of agriculture, we can now grow and have access to vegetables out of season, too.

Our bodies naturally need these seasonal vegetables at the time they are grown so that we can be in tune with nature. You will find that you feel more satisfied if you eat seasonally. That's partly because the nutritional value is higher in a vegetable that is grown in its natural habitat and harvested at maturity, rather than some time before it's ripe so it can be packaged and transported long distances. It's also because our bodies need different foods according to the seasons. Somehow Mother Nature figured out how to supply us best.

A salad, for example, can be very satisfying in the summer but less so in the middle of winter. Fruit, too, can be too cold to enjoy in January, but nothing is more refreshing in the middle of July. On the other hand, a hot stew is too heavy on a hot day but the perfect comfort food when there's snow on the ground outside.

→ What sustains our energy for the long haul is complex carbohydrates.

→ You will find that you feel more satisfied if you eat seasonally.

→ You can get your necessary fat and protein from plant-based foods too!

THE NURTURE OF GREEN

One subset of the vegetable kingdom deserves special mention: leafy greens and other green vegetables. These foods are so powerful and contribute so much to so many aspects of our well-being and health, I call them super foods. Here's why:

Green vegetables assist in elimination and detoxification, necessary processes for optimum health. When it comes to eliminating toxins from the body, they are the hardworking liver's greatest ally.

Leafy greens have especially high antioxidant levels (carotenoids, beta carotene, and vitamin E), linking them to improved heart health and, according to many studies, endowing them with anti-cancer properties. They are an excellent source of vitamin A and a good source of vitamin C (the darker the leaves, the more vitamin A they contain). Many greens are known for their mineral content, especially iron, calcium, and magnesium, as well as folate, riboflavin (B2), and vitamin K. And of course they are high in fiber (which contributes to intestinal health and the sustenance of energy levels). Often greens require little cooking, which means they can be consumed in their most nutritious states, in many cases raw or only lightly cooked.

There's more: Eating greens helps to balance the bacteria in the intestinal tract. This in turn helps us absorb our foods better, which allows us to get more satisfaction from less food.

Lastly, greens have an alkalizing effect on the blood, which reduces inflammation, a major cause of illness. And just imagine this: *A whole pound of broccoli is only 130 kcal.*

Incorporating more green vegetables into your diet is the first step you can take to better health and toward mastering your appetite. When you give them the chance, you'll find that greens are so satisfying to eat, they can do wonders for balancing your weight by providing low-calorie meals, preventing excessive eating from false hunger, and lessening sweet cravings.

◐

The abundance of green vegetable choices available today always amazes me. It could be because I grew up without much access to leafy greens, or because I always notice how much satisfaction they add to a meal—even if they don't add many calories. I cannot stress enough how important leafy greens and green vegetables are to gaining more nourishment (both the *feeling* of satiation and the *fact* of nutrition) from your food, and to being able to eat more bulk without a lot of calories—two essential aspects of mastering your appetite.

TYPES OF LEAFY GREENS

Arugula: This has a peppery spicy flavor. It's great both raw and slightly wilted in a hot dish.

Belgian Endive: This has a dense, elongated egg shape and is about five inches long, with whitish-yellow crunchy leaves and a bitter taste. It is often mixed raw with milder greens but also very nice cooked or thrown on the barbecue.

Bok Choy: One of the oldest greens, this has been cultivated for at least 1500 years. It comes both in a baby version and with large crunchy leaves. In its larger incarnation, the stem is white or pale green with slightly wavy, light-green leaves. The baby version looks more like the leaf version of an endive. Bok Choy is great for sautéing or stir-frying with other vegetables. It is often used in Chinese cooking. "Pak Choi" is an alternate spelling for the same vegetable.

Boston or Bibb: This is a delicious head lettuce with a soft buttery texture. The leaves are loose, succulent, and almost oily, green or brown-red on the outside and creamy white toward the middle.

Collards: These have large, flat, dark-green leaves that look like a fan. Along with kale, collards are among the most nutritious of the greens and are delicious when cooked.

Curly Endive: Sometimes called chicory, this is sharply flavored, crisp, and curly with dark-green leaves on the outside and lighter green leaves on the inside, which is also more tender. It's a good cooking green.

Kale: This is usually flat with frilled edges or very curly like oversized parsley. You can also find dinosaur kale, which has narrower and longer leaves. Kale is very dark and dense in texture, making it delicious when cooked in with a soup or sautéed on its own. Blanching and steaming is always an option for the dark leafy greens (and see my recipe for marinated kale in the Cooking Basics chapter).

Head Lettuce: This is a general term for lettuce that is harvested as a full head rather than as individual leaves. There are many varieties; it can be reddish or green. The leaves can be waxy with curly edges, flat-looking like a tree leaf, or even frilly.

Mâche: This wonderful light small-leafed green has a buttery taste. It works well as a topping on fish or vegetable dishes, but it almost disappears if mixed with other greens. It can be grown in cold weather, so if you're lucky you might find it freshly harvested at a farmers' market well into the fall.

Mesclun: This is a general term from France for salad mixes that combine leaf lettuce (harvested young) with other smaller greens such as arugula, dandelion, or endive.

Mizuna: This mustard green of Japanese origin has a white thin stalk and a fringed, deeply cut leaf. Its mild flavor is perfect for salads. If cooked, it needs very little; just mixing it with something hot is enough.

Radicchio: This ruby-red little head with white veins has a bitter taste. It's a colorful mixer with other milder greens but also holds up its flavor very well when sautéed.

Romaine: This head lettuce used in Caesar salads supposedly got its name from the Romans. Loose and upright, it has thick, elongated leaves with heavy stiff midribs.

Spinach: This was the first leafy green I learned about as a kid because of Popeye. It comes both in a baby form, which is good raw in salads, and with longer leaves that are great for cooking. Even though it is mildly flavored, it does belong to the family of bitter greens. (Do note that spinach belongs to the nightshade family of plants, which can cause inflammation of the joints in those who have arthritis; it can also block iron absorption, so is best avoided by those who are anemic.)

Sprouts: Although not a leafy green, these deserve a mention because they are a great add-on to any salad due to their crunch and their high nutritional value.

Tatsoi: This small, dark, spoon-shaped green leaf has a unique, mild taste. It's delicious raw in salads and can also be lightly cooked.

Watercress: This very nutritious little dark green with medium to small leaves on stems has a peppery taste. It's great both raw and cooked.

THE MIGHTY CRUCIFEROUS: QUEEN OF THE VEGGIES

The cruciferous vegetables are broccoli and its family, which includes cauliflower, Brussels sprouts, cabbage, and kale. Also referred to as the cabbage family, these highly nutritious vegetables have long been used in stews and soups, as well as fermented and pickled. For several years now, they have been the most popular fresh vegetables on the plate. They are best eaten just slightly steamed or sautéed, and they mix well with other vegetables. Cabbage is often used raw in salads, marinated, sautéed, or cooked into soups.

The cruciferous vegetables are very high in vitamin A, C, and K; folic acid; and minerals. They are dense and high in fiber, hence a good food choice for mastering your appetite. From a health perspective, they are believed to contain anti-cancer properties because of their antioxidants and phytochemicals. Like the leafy greens they have a detoxifying effect, and they help in fighting carcinogens and free radicals. They also protect against anti-oxidative stress on our cell system, which makes them powerful in fighting disease and the effects of aging.

The cruciferous vegetables can be hard to digest, especially when eaten raw, due to their dense cell walls—but a quick, slight steam or sauté is enough to make them more digestible. If you have thyroid issues, you won't want to skip this light cooking, as eating raw cruciferous vegetables can worsen thyroid functions.

It is important to chew these vegetables well in order to avoid bloating and indigestion. So wait to blame it on the vegetables if you don't do too well in the beginning. Give them another try; they are good for you and help you feel satisfied for hours. Practice chewing!

Of all the vegetables, these two groups—cruciferous and leafy greens—give you the most fiber and nourishment, which lead to greater satiation and mastery of your appetite.

> → Green vegetables assist in elimination and detoxification, necessary processes for optimum health.

> → Choose vegetables from the cruciferous group and leafy greens for maximum satiation and mastery of your appetite.

ONIONS: FOOD & MEDICINE

You may have heard the saying, "If you eat onions every day, you'll live to be a hundred." While this is not a scientifically proven statement, the onion family has received a lot of well-deserved attention among scientists.

Onions belong to the same family as garlic, leeks, chives, scallions, and shallots. For many years, they have been used for their medicinal properties; they have a healing effect on colds, coughs, and asthmatic conditions. Onions are rich in fructo-oligosaccharides, which is essential for our cells and for balancing the bacteria in the colon. In fact, it helps remove heavy metals and parasites from our intestines and is therefore an important food in our daily detoxification.

Onions are also a good source of chromium, an important trace mineral that helps with blood sugar balance. They improve glucose tolerance and lower insulin levels. When our blood sugar levels stabilize, so do our insulin levels and, with that, our hunger signals. Chromium deficiency is common because chromium gets depleted when we eat simple carbohydrates like sugar and baked flour products. You could take a supplement to add chromium, but consider adding more cooked onions to your meals instead—they offer so much more.

Onions contain high levels of vitamin C, calcium, magnesium, phosphorus, and potassium. Also found in onion is the antioxidant quercetin, a natural antihistamine and anti-inflammatory agent. All of this makes onion one of the most powerful anti-cancer foods.

Onions range in taste and can be both spicy and sweet. The sweetness of cooked onions (cook them long enough and they "caramelize") can be very nourishing and a boon for those with a sweet tooth because they help master cravings for sugary foods. Raw onion—especially the sweeter varieties—can be a delicious addition to salads when sliced thinly; but beware the very real result of eating onions raw: onion breath!

THE ROOTS OF NURTURE

Root vegetables are mostly sweet, but some are slightly bitter or spicy. They are all rich in fiber, full of nutrients, and great for satisfying your hunger.

What often happens is that we don't get enough sweet foods in our daily diet, so we end up going for sweetened foods and dessert instead.

This may be news: You can satisfy your sweet tooth by adding more wholegrain, sweet roots, and cooked onion to your meals.

◎

For centuries, roots have been regarded as peasant food, hearty and dependable; because they store well, they were also the only vegetable available during the winter months in the cold climates of the north. Sweet and loaded with energy, they're rich in comfort. And many roots have traditionally been used for medicinal purposes for thousands of years.

Root vegetables and winter squash are good sources of vitamins A, B and C, as well as niacin, potassium, copper, magnesium, folic acid, iron, phosphorus, and pantothenic acid (the values vary for each). Those deeper in color contain health-promoting antioxidants and phytochemicals—for example, beta carotene is found in deep-orange carrots, sweet potatoes, and pumpkin.

Also a good source of fiber, roots are relatively low in calories. This makes them excellent for mastering your appetite and feeling satiated from your meal at the same time. They also provide a good source of complex glucose. They have gained a bad reputation for being high in sugar, but several studies have confirmed that a diet based on wholegrain and vegetables, including roots, can be more beneficial for diabetics than the commonly recommended diet plan.

Another finding has shown that the glycemic index in carrots is high in a laboratory environment but that when eaten and digested in the body, it's in fact low. The fiber in the carrots slows down the absorption time, and as a result our blood-sugar levels remain stable. As a reminder, this is one of the major clues to mastering your appetite—and your health. Just think of how you feel when eating a sweet cooked root vegetable such as carrot, beet, sweet potato, parsnip, or turnip. Full with comfort and nurture—and, of course, nutrients.

To be a "true" root, a vegetable needs to grow underground and play the role of a root for the greens above ground: absorbing moisture and nutrients from the ground. Generally, this term is used for any part of a plant that grows underground.

Root vegetables are: beets, burdock, daikon, carrots, horseradish, radishes, rutabagas, parsnips, salsify, and turnips. The "tubers"—sweet potatoes, yams, and various other potato family members —also grow underground but aren't technically root vegetables since they aren't the plant's root; similarly, garlic and onions ("bulbs") are non-root vegetables that grow underground.

◑

And then we have the gourds, which include pumpkin, winter squash, and all the warty, odd-shaped decorative fruit that simply go by the name "gourd." Gourds originated in the western hemisphere and were being consumed by man at least 5,000 years ago. Winter squashes—including butternut, acorn, and spaghetti squash—are characterized by firm flesh and thick skin. They typically require longer cooking than other vegetables. For some of them, the cooked skin can be eaten, but most people prefer to carve out the "meat" only and dispose of the skin. Either way, they are sweet, satisfying, and nice to add to a meal. But I would caution against making roots and squashes the main part of your meal; they can end up providing too much starch if eaten in excess. The result would be that you crave more sugar and sweetness afterwards instead of feeling satisfied.

Gourds keep well in a cool dark place for up to several months and don't need to be refrigerated. Root vegetables can also be stored for a long period of time—best in the fridge, as some of their vitamin content is sensitive to light.

GRAINS: THE DAILY GRAIN, NOT THE DAILY BREAD

In the typical daily diet of many, bread is considered the grain of the day, and cooked wholegrain got lost for years if not generations. Most of us know by now that bread—especially white bread—is considered a "bad carbohydrate," but we also know that bread is one of those hard-to-resist foods that are shunned by diets and binged on when the opportunity is there.

Thankfully, cooked wholegrain dishes are making a strong comeback, and so is the understanding that white bread is not the same as wholegrain bread. I also want to add that cooked wholegrain is not the same as white rice. Confused? It just comes down to what we've been saying all along: *All carbohydrates are not created equal.*

◎

Wholegrain is one of those essential foods that have been modified over the years and, in the process, became filler foods instead of the nutritional powerhouse that they really are. For a time, the novelty and expense of processing meant that the whiter the bread, the more desired and valuable. Now it's the processed white bread that is cheap, and good dense wholegrain bread has gone up in price.

Still today, however, most people think of grain as synonymous with bread, and bread as synonymous with empty carbs—so they try to limit their intake of grain or avoid it altogether. I believe strongly that the Atkins diet committed a real health *faux pas* by telling us to say no to carbohydrates. As a result, so many people with the best intentions of improving their health have lost out on the important and essential glucose that comes from the complex carbohydrates in wholegrain foods. Today the similarly carb-averse Paleo diet is encouraging countless people to lose out on the complex glucose the brain needs for cognitive ability. Remember that the mood-enhancing hormone serotonin is found in carbohydrates; concurrent with the vilification of carbs in popular diets, low serotonin levels have caused an increase in depression and in our general inability to be focused and calm on a day-to-day basis.

I will not judge whether the Atkins or Paleo diets are 100% wrong in their approach, but I do want to point to a range of health problems that are connected to high levels of animal fat and animal protein, such as higher inflammation and kidney problems. Essentially, I believe we need to learn how to eat from a sustainable perspective and understand which foods feed us and which don't. There are many healthful qualities wholegrain can contribute to our daily food choices.

Growing up in Denmark, I was fed dark rye breads and heavier grains like barley in cooked dishes.

White flour was reserved for pastries. This meant that white flour was in the same category as refined sugar: something to indulge in once in a while, in small quantities, as a special treat. I believe this is the healthiest approach. The fact is: We crave the carbohydrates in grains, but we need to avoid the refined variety. If we want to live in a balanced, sustainable way and also master our appetites while feeling nourished, cooked wholegrain needs to find its way back onto our plates in appropriate proportions.

◎

The desire for comfort food gets the better of us all on a regular basis. This occurs particularly when we are stressed, sad, mad, or tired—all good reasons for needing comfort. One of the most popular comfort foods is pasta—a refined flour product, like white bread, that has little true nourishment to offer.

Fortunately, if you love pasta you now have plenty of healthier options: wholegrain pasta can certainly be part of a healthy diet, as long as it's eaten with a lot of fiber-rich vegetables (and stay away from the heavy sauces). Pasta made from wholegrain other than wheat is also much more readily available every year. My personal favorite is brown rice pasta because it's gluten free.

So what happens during the refining process that turns a wonderful food—wholegrain—into a nutrition-free echo of its former self? All refined flour was wholegrain once upon a time, before the outer shell was removed, leaving only the inner kernel. Too bad: It's precisely in these outer layers of the germ and the bran that most of the nutrients are found.

When grain is refined and the fiber (and nutrition) is removed, eating it causes a faster spike in blood sugar levels. Although grain is a complex carbohydrate, after it's refined it acts like a simple one— with little nutritional content, all it produces is a momentary burst of energy followed by a crash. We wind up hungry shortly after eating and reach for seconds—that's why I call refined wheat flour products the "more-more food."

This is not the case with cooked wholegrain. Cooked wholegrain is very satisfying for several reasons: It is still high in fiber, its higher nutrient levels are intact, it promotes steady blood-sugar levels that eliminate the spike-and-crash of refined grains—and, since it increases levels of the feel-good hormone serotonin, it has comforting values. *A meal that incorporates cooked wholegrain helps you master your appetite far better in the long run than will a piece of bread.*

◑

Because of the higher fiber content, some people can have a difficult time digesting wholegrain when they first introduce it into their diets. This was why people started refining grain in the first place: to make it easier to digest. But there is a better, easier way to render wholegrain more digestible: *Chew better.* Human saliva contains digestive enzymes that are needed to break down complex carbohydrates; if you experience bloating after eating wholegrain, it could be because you didn't chew well.

But what about gluten intolerance and sensitivity? If you get bloated after eating bread even if it's wholegrain and you chew it well, it is very possibly because of the gluten that is found in wheat. Whether or not you have been diagnosed with

Celiac disease or gluten intolerance, if you consistently have a negative reaction to wheat, you would probably do best to simply avoid it!

Partly due to the high incidence of gluten sensitivity, I mostly suggest avoiding bread altogether and focusing instead on cooked grains, with an emphasis on gluten-free grain like brown and wild rice, oats, and millet. If you can tolerate gluten but have a negative reaction to wheat (which is very common and may have to do with the chemically assisted harvesting practices of commercial wheat) you can still try barley, rye, and possibly kamut, farro, and spelt. These last three grains are ancient strains in the same family as wheat, but many who are intolerant to wheat are not intolerant to them. You might also experiment with whole wheat-berries—also known as einkorn. Just try small amounts, chew well, and see how you feel.

Rice is completely gluten free and is the most ubiquitous example of cooked grain. But be aware: There's a difference between white and brown rice. White rice is like white flour: It's been refined and the bran part has been removed to make it easier to digest. Just as with other grains, this process causes white rice to have a higher glycemic index and lower fiber content—which make it less nourishing and less satisfying to eat.

◑

When we say that wholegrain has a "low glycemic index," this means that what makes these carbohydrates complex (fiber) causes the glucose from them to be digested and absorbed slower—which means it enters the bloodstream slower. This provides a more stable and sustaining energy for longer and helps you master your appetite. Wholegrain also aids in balancing our mood swings by keeping steady blood-sugar levels, while increasing the efficiency of our brain functions. Wholegrain is, indeed, brain food.

Also, the complex carbohydrates of wholegrain contain beneficial phytonutrients, vitamins, and minerals. When whole, the germ or "heart" of the kernel is still intact with its essential vitamin B, iron, and zinc.

But the thing that is probably least known about wholegrain is this: Even though it's primarily a carbohydrate, *wholegrain contains good levels of protein, too.* This is probably why grain has been such a stable part of the food supply for so many centuries.

WHOLEGRAIN FACTS AT A GLANCE:

- Grains are the seeds of plants. When whole, they include the bran, germ, and endosperm, all of which contain valuable nutrients.

- Wholegrain is rich in fiber. Fiber makes you feel full and satisfies your appetite for several hours. It also slows down the absorption of glucose into your bloodstream, so your energy is longer lasting.

- Fiber in your diet assists in the elimination of waste and toxins from your intestines; it's also needed for good digestion.

- Eating wholegrain aids in balancing your mood and sharpens your mental focus because it increases serotonin and because brains need carbohydrates for cognitive ability.

- You can add wholegrain to your diet as a cooked grain or by choosing wholegrain bread (make sure it says "wholegrain," not just whole wheat).

- Brown rice, barley, oats, rye, wild rice, millet, and quinoa (also considered a protein) are probably the most accessible cooked grains; all are great choices. Whole rolled oats or steel-cut oats and rye for a hot breakfast cereal like oatmeal are a better choice than the instant stuff. I recommend choosing whole dark all-rye and sprouted wholegrain breads over those made with refined wheat flour.

- Wholegrain has been shown to reduce the risk of heart disease by decreasing cholesterol levels, blood pressure, and blood coagulation.

- Wholegrain has been found to reduce the risks of many types of cancer.

- Wholegrain has also been shown to help regulate blood glucose, which is important for all of us but especially for those living with diabetes.

- Studies have shown that people who consume wholegrain consistently weigh less than those who don't. Surprise, right?

WHOLE & GRAINY CHOICES

Barley: A great alternative to rice, this can also be used as a breakfast cereal and added to soups and stews. High in fiber, it helps to metabolize fats, cholesterol, and carbohydrates.

Brown rice: This flexible grain can be added to many dishes or eaten on its own. It is also used for making gluten-free pasta. Much higher in nutrient levels than white rice, it contains not only the fiber that helps to lower cholesterol but also vitamin B and high levels of manganese, selenium, magnesium, and tryptophan. These vitamins and minerals may add to the reasons that people who eat brown rice on a regular basis feel calmer and more satisfied.

Buckwheat: This is technically not a grain, but it's commonly used in place of grains or in combination with them. It is unrelated to wheat and is in fact gluten free—plus it's loaded with protein and high in amino acids, and it is known to stabilize blood sugar and reduce hypertension. It can be substituted for wheat when making crêpes or pancakes, and while it won't work in place of wheat in conventional bread recipes, there are good recipes available for buckwheat-based bread.

Millet: A nutty, gluten-free grain, it is both low in glycemic load and high in magnesium, manganese, thiamin, niacin, folate, and protein. It's delicious as a savory grain dish mixed with vegetables or as a breakfast cereal.

Oats: These provide a good source of complex carbohydrates and soluble fiber, especially rolled or steel-cut for oatmeal. One half-cup serving of oats supplies about nine grams of fiber. Though oats themselves are gluten free, they are often processed alongside wheat; if you have Celiac disease or a severe intolerance, you'll want to look for oats that are labeled "gluten free."

Quinoa: This ancient seed in the family of leafy greens is, like buckwheat, not technically a grain, though we tend to use it as one. It is not only high in protein, it is a complete protein, which is not the case with true grains. It was the staple of the Incas—a food for warriors—with its high levels of nutrients such as magnesium, potassium, zinc, vitamin E, riboflavin, copper, Omega-3 fatty acids, and more iron than grains. Basically, this is one of the great superfoods. It is also gluten free.

Rye: This binds with water quickly and gives a feeling of fullness and satiety—it's an excellent choice for mastering your appetite. Cooking rye as a grain or eating all wholegrain rye bread (not wheat with rye added) helps you lose weight. A cup of rye cereal alone provides 17% of the daily value for fiber. It is also rich in magnesium, which is an important mineral used by more than 300 enzymes to do their work in our body, including the enzymes that affect our use of glucose and insulin secretion. This makes an all-rye bread a better choice than wheat bread for people with diabetes and for anyone who wants to master their weight and their appetite. Rye bread is the bread of choice for my Scandinavian heritage and I grew up eating it instead of wheat bread. Luckily it is now more accessible in stores in America, normally packaged and already thinly sliced. In most stores, it is sold as German rye bread and resembles pumpernickel bread.

→ You can satisfy your sweet tooth by adding more wholegrain, sweet roots, and even cooked onion to your meals.

→ A meal that incorporates cooked wholegrain helps you master your appetite far better in the long run than will a piece of bread.

PROTEIN: WHAT, HOW & WHY

Most of us have learned that protein comes from animal sources and that we have to eat protein in every meal because it's essential for building muscle—which is why the tendency to eat a lot of meat is especially pronounced in body-builders. But while we certainly all need protein, we don't need as much as is often assumed. The official recommendation is .36 grams per pound of body weight per day, far less than most Americans eat. So a 150-pound person will need about 55 grams of protein per day. A 4-ounce piece of fish has about 24 grams of protein in it, so you can see how easy it is to get enough.

Additionally we get protein from a wide variety of foods, not just animal products—did you know that there's protein in all food, even broccoli? In this section we'll address the importance of protein and the relative benefits of its different sources.

The heart of protein: amino acids

Protein molecules are made up of amino acids, which control the expansion and contraction of muscles and are considered the builders of cells and muscle tissue. They are essential to maintaining the health of our cells, blood, hair, skin, and bones, and they are important to the digestive process and the immune system, since they are also what form the antibodies that fight infections.

There are several amino acids—some say 20, some say 22—that are necessary for our bodies to function properly. Many of these can be synthesized by the human body, so we don't need to worry so much about getting them from food: These are called the "dispensable" amino acids and they include alanine, aspartic acid, asparagine, glutamic acid and serine.

There are, however, nine amino acids that we need to get from our food every day because the human body is unable to synthesize them on its own. These are the "essential" amino acids: phenylalanine, valine, threonine, tryptophan, methionine, leucine, isoleucine, lysine, and histidine.

One reason people tend to identify meat, dairy, and soy as good sources of protein is that, in fact, there is only a short list of foods that can provide *all* of the essential amino acids—it includes meat, poultry, fish, eggs, dairy, soy, and quinoa. As a result, you may have heard these foods referred to as "complete proteins."

But foods that contain only some of the essential amino acids—including vegetables, legumes, and grains—can still contribute heartily to your protein intake. What this means is that if you are vegan, you don't have to live on quinoa alone! During the digestive process, protein molecules are broken down into their parts—the amino acids—that are then absorbed into the body, which at that point doesn't care where the amino acids come from, as long as they're all there. You can create a meal that contains a complete supply of protein simply by combining a variety of foods.

Animal or vegetable?

Plants make proteins from minerals they absorb in the soil; grass-fed animals, in turn, get all of their protein from the plants they eat. In other words, many animals do not get any of their protein from eating other animals.

If you choose to include meat in your diet, limiting it to grass-fed and free-grazing animal sources is better both for your health and for the animals. Factory-farmed (non-grazing) animals are raised primarily on corn, which makes their meat fatty—good for sales! But the corn-based feed is hard for them to digest since it's not part of their natural diet. They end up with diseases, for which they are given antibiotics. Also, the corn they are fed is often from GMO sources, which is not healthy for them, or for us.

The quality of the meat we choose also affects how satisfied we feel; while grass-fed meat is lower in saturated fat, it's also higher in muscle mass, which fills us up. Additionally, supermarket meat is pumped up with water and nitrates, which is not only unhealthy, it makes the meat less satisfying—and that prompts us to eat more of it.

Eggs offer a good source of protein that is more easily digested than the meat of the animal it would turn into. But factory-farmed chickens suffer as much as cows from mistreatment, poor feeding and disease, and they too are raised on antibiotics. As with all animal products, the health of the animal becomes the health value of your food; choose only GMO-free, organic, free-range, antibiotic-free eggs.

Fish is healthier than meats from land animals because its fat is higher in Omega-3 fatty acids (more on those in the next section). And, of course, it is one of the "complete proteins."

I want to stress that it's possible to get all the protein you need without eating meat, or eating very little of it. Legumes like beans, peas, and lentils provide as many grams of protein per ounce as chicken. Combine them with vegetables and whole grains, and you can get all nine essential amino acids without eating any animal products.

Additionally, while the fats in meat and fish make us feel more immediately satisfied, the fiber in legumes can give us a longer-lasting and healthier feeling of satisfaction, while we also feel lighter because legumes and vegetables are easier to digest.

For your overall health, I recommend relying more on legumes than on meat for your protein (and of the animal proteins, choosing fish over other sources when you can); not only are plants healthier for you, the negative environmental effects of meat production—including its impact on global warming—are well known.

Legumes
Many think of legumes—beans, lentils and peas—as fattening foods, or as foods that cause gas and discomfort. It's true that legumes are very filling, but that doesn't mean they're fattening. If you find

that you feel gassy after eating legumes, how you cook them might be part of the problem. Always cook legumes without salt (you can add some to taste after they are cooked). Also, make sure to chew well. For some, the addition of garlic, onions, or kombu can help with digestion, while others find that onion too can cause gas. Experiment, and see what works for you.

Current high-protein diets like the Paleo diet discourage the eating of legumes, but studies have found that they promote weight loss because of their low glycemic index, which means they help balance blood-glucose and insulin levels—one of the keys to mastering your appetite and your weight.

> → There are nine essential amino acids (proteins) that we need to get from our food every day because the human body is unable to synthesize them on its own.

> → While only a few foods contain all of the essential amino acids—meat, poultry, fish, eggs, dairy, soy, and quinoa (the "complete proteins")—you can easily get them all from a vegan diet by mixing various vegetables, legumes, and grains.

PROTEIN, DIGESTION & APPETITE

Protein is important to balancing your weight for three reasons: First, it slows down the digestive process, since protein-rich foods take longer to move from the stomach to the intestines. This can make you feel fuller for longer. Second, protein helps avoid quick rises in blood-sugar levels, and this stabilizes your hunger. Third, the body uses up more energy (more calories) to digest protein. But the important thing to remember is that all of these weight-loss benefits are equally available from plant-based protein and can be fully accessed when you eat far less meat than the average American—or even no meat at all.

Why less (animal) protein is more

The original meats in our ancestors" diets were wild game and birds, fish and waterfowl. The domestication of animals like sheep, goats, and cattle became important for our evolution, but today we tend to eat mostly factory-farmed beef and chicken, both higher in acidity than our heritage meats. Acidic foods like meat increase inflammation in our bodies, which leaves us struggling with out-of-control hunger and weight gain, as well as disease.

When there is excess acidity in our bodies, it gets neutralized by calcium. The greatest source of calcium is the skeleton, so diets high in protein—especially from high-acid animal sources—can lead to calcium loss, also known as osteoporosis.

The whole point of eating better is to improve your health while feeling more satisfied from each meal—which in turn will help you to master not only your appetite, but also your weight. Basically we need protein in our meals, but we need to eat it in the right proportion to vegetables and starches.

Reminder: My recommendation for a balanced plate is: ½ low-starch vegetables, ¼ starch (wholegrain or root vegetables), and ¼ protein.

DAIRY

To master your appetite I don't recommend including dairy in your daily food choices. Here's why:

Dairy sugars can cause a rise in insulin, which can lead to blood-sugar imbalances, one of the causes of increased appetite and the desire to binge.

Dairy can also become a trigger food for overeating. It's difficult to stop eating it once you start, because so many dairy-based foods offer a "bliss-point" combination of ingredients: With cheese it's fat, sugar, and salt; with ice cream it's that special combination of sweetness and fat that might even bring back unconscious memories of mother's milk (which is actually sweeter than cow's milk).

Low-fat and nonfat dairy products, though marketed as foods that support weight loss, are in fact detrimental to mastering your appetite. Why? Because when you remove the fat, you're left with the sugar!

I go more into the health reasons for avoiding dairy in my online program, but for our purposes here, I'll just offer this suggestion: If you don't want to give up dairy completely, make sure any dairy products you consume are made with whole milk, and stick with those from free-range, growth hormone– and antibiotic-free cows, goats, and sheep. The healthiest dairy food would be unpasteurized raw milk, because it still contains all the naturally present enzymes and nutrients, but in most states it can only be bought legally directly from the farm.

→ If you choose to include meat in your diet, limiting it to grass-fed and free-grazing animal sources is better both for your health and for the animals.

→ As with all animal products, the health of the animal becomes the health value of your food; choose organic, antibiotic-free, free-range eggs.

→ A balanced plate will contain ½ low-starch vegetables, ¼ starch (wholegrain or root vegetables), and ¼ protein.

THE SKINNY ON FATS

About a decade ago, Americans received a message from scientists and nutritionists to eliminate fat from our diets. This was one of the most misunderstood and miscommunicated food-related messages of our time.

There was an essential oversight in these communications: the difference between good fats, not-so-good fats, and ugly fats. The message "Eat fat-free!" implies that all fats are created equal, but they aren't: The truth is that some fats should be avoided completely, some are OK to consume in small quantities, and some are in fact both beneficial and necessary, not just for overall health but also for weight loss and mastering your appetite.

Fats and appetite mastery

Healthy fats help us feel satisfied by the food we eat. One reason for this is simple: Fats help food taste good, and tasty food is more satisfying. But there is another, more important reason, which has to do with the way our bodies absorb nutrients from the food we eat.

Vitamins and minerals are either water or fat-soluble, which means that if we don't include fat in our diets, our bodies aren't able to absorb the nutrients from a meal—in essence, we're depriving our bodies of some of the value of our food. We're also slowing down the process of digestion when we add healthy fats, which help us stay full for longer.

Have you ever noticed how easy it is to eat an entire bag of fat-free cookies? Plenty of foods are naturally fat free, but whenever you eat a fat-free version of a food that would normally contain fat (like ice cream or cookies), you can be sure that you're eating a food product stripped of most of its nutrition; and since it's less satisfying, no matter how much of it you eat you'll still be left craving the real thing. You'll also find there is more sugar than needed in fat-free foods. This is because the lack of taste from the missing fats is made up for with added sugar.

It's far better to consume some fat and to do so in an informed way. This means increasing your intake of good fats, limiting your intake of "not-so-good" fats, and avoiding ugly fats entirely.

> → The message "Eat fat-free!" implies that all fats are created equal, but they aren't: Some fats are fine to eat in small quantities and some are actually beneficial to overall health and promote weight loss.

> → When we add healthy fats to our diets, we slow down the process of digestion, which helps us stay full for longer.

THE GOOD, THE NOT-SO-GOOD & THE UGLY

The Ugly: Fats to avoid
Ugly" fat—also called "trans fat"—is a coagulated, hard-to-digest vegetable fat produced by a process

of hydrogenation. It was developed primarily to increase the shelf life of packaged foods (we've all heard about how a Twinkie will never go stale). Our bodies do not recognize this type of fat as food, and they simply don't know what to do with it. As a result, it clogs up our system, from the intestines to the arteries. Trans fat raises total and LDL (bad) cholesterol levels while also lowering HDL (good) cholesterol levels. It's a true health hazard that's fortunately being phased out due to the increased education of consumers—and, in some cases, due to regulation. But you still need to beware its presence in packaged goods.

It is now legally required for food manufacturers to list trans fat on their labels, but there's a catch: If a product contains less than .05 grams of it per serving, the requirement does not apply. This means that it's easy to eat quite a bit of trans fat without realizing it, just by eating several cookies, for example (where one cookie = one serving) from a company that is taking advantage of this loophole. Of course, if you stick to unpackaged, unprocessed foods, you don't have to worry about ever accidentally eating this "ugly fat."

If you do eat packaged food (including butter substitutes), always check labels for "trans fat" or its other name, "partially hydrogenated oil." And bear in mind that fully hydrogenated oil, which will be listed as "hydrogenated oil," is still a very unhealthy fat, but it is chemically different from trans fat and is slightly less ugly.

The "Not-so-good": Fats to consume with care

Naturally occurring fats (as opposed to processed trans fat) break down into two main groups: saturated and unsaturated. To make it all more confusing, unsaturated fats can be either polyunsaturated or monounsaturated. Each type has a different health value. I'll go into each type with a bit more detail below, but if you want a rule of thumb first, here's how these fats stack up:

(1) Monounsaturated fat (higher health benefit)

(2) Polyunsaturated fat (moderate health benefit)

(3) Saturated fat (least healthy, to be consumed only in small quantities)

Saturated fats. These fats come almost exclusively from animal sources—meat, poultry, and dairy—and are considered the least healthy natural fats because they clog arteries and directly raise total and LDL (bad) cholesterol levels. The exception to this rule is coconut oil, which is a plant-derived saturated fat that actually is shown to lower cholesterol and increase overall health. After years of being shunned, it is now promoted as a healthy choice. (I recommend trying it in recipes that call for butter or margarine.) Fish and eggs also contain saturated fats, but these are lower in saturated fats than other meat and dairy products and they contain essential Omega-3 fatty acids (more on those below).

Monounsaturated fats and *ploy-unsaturated* fats are two types of unsaturated fatty acids. They are derived from vegetables and plants.

Monounsaturated fats become liquid at room temperature and solidify at cold temperatures. Preferred to oils higher in polyunsaturated fat, these mono fats come from oils made of olives; nuts like almond, walnut, and peanut; and canola, sunflower and avocado. Studies have shown that these fats can lower LDL (bad) cholesterol and maintain HDL (good) cholesterol. Canola oil is often from genetically modified sources, though, so unless you can find a GMO-free brand, I don't tend to recommend it.

Polyunsaturated fats are found in sesame, safflower, grape-seed, corn, cottonseed, and soybean oils. This type of fat has also been shown to reduce levels of LDL cholesterol, but too much of it can also lower your HDL cholesterol. They are liquid both in the fridge and at room temperature. In general I suggest avoiding corn, canola, and soybean oil completely because they are so often from GMO sources.

Cooking with oil

There are important things to consider when cooking with oil. Some oils can be used for high-heat cooking, while others have lower smoke points. It's important that you check the smoke points, because when you heat oils and fats above their smoke point, they become carcinogens. In general, the process of refining an oil will raise its smoke-point; but as is often the case, the process of refining oil also depletes it of some of its nutritional value.

My favorite oils to use in cooking are untoasted sesame oil and coconut oil because of their added health benefits. Sesame oil contains phytosterols, plant-derived fatty compounds that resemble cholesterol in their chemistry and function. This means they reduce cholesterol absorption into your blood by as much as 60 percent, according to studies. Coconut oil, though a saturated fat, has a very high amount of medium-chain fatty acids (or triglycerides), which help the body burn stored fat.

Here are my recommended healthy-choice oils broken down by function:

Baking: coconut oil or nut oils

Salad dressing, grain mixes, and to drizzle on top of your food before serving: Cold pressed, extra-virgin (organic) olive oil; hemp, flax, and pumpkin seed oil

Low-heat cooking: Untoasted sesame oil, coconut oil, nut oils, and olive oil

High-heat cooking: coconut oil, untoasted sesame oil, grape-seed oil, safflower oil

The "good" fats: Omega-3 fatty acids
You have probably heard of Omega-3 fatty acids and their myriad health benefits. Omega-3 is a polyunsaturated fat, but it falls into the "great for you" category and is actually essential to a healthy

diet. That's why you see it packaged in supplements—but you can also get the Omega-3 acids you need from well-chosen, satisfying food.

Some signs of Omega-3 deficiency include cracked nails; constipation; dry skin, hair, and mouth; fatigue; forgetfulness; immune weakness; and lack of endurance and motivation. Many health conditions are linked to insufficient intake of Omega-3, including: acne, allergies, Alzheimer's, arthritis, ADD, autoimmune diseases, breast cancer and cysts, dementia, depression, dermatitis, diabetes, eczema, heart disease, high blood pressure, hyperactivity, hypertension, immune disorders, IBS, inflammatory conditions, kidney dysfunction, learning difficulties, menopausal symptoms, MS, pregnancy complications, psoriasis, stroke, and vascular disease. In Scandinavia, multiple studies have shown the huge importance of Omega-3, especially for brain development and general health. In addition to all their other benefits, Omega-3 fats are excellent tools for mastering your appetite and for losing weight, since they help burn the fat stored in our bodies and around our organs.

Omega-3 fatty acids are critical to keeping our entire body, cells, tissue, and organs functioning. They are naturally anti-inflammatory and help positively affect both our cholesterol and insulin levels (as I explained in the section on sugar, maintaining insulin levels is crucial to your general health but also to your appetite and your weight). And they are crucial for our brain health, too: Two-thirds of the brain is composed of fatty acids, affecting everything from our thoughts to our moods—both of which can help in the mastery of your appetite.

As if that isn't enough, Omega-3 has been found to help fight depression, and I think we can all agree that feeling down often leads to making unhealthy food choices and to overeating.

Good sources of Omega-3 acids are oily and cold-water fish; flax, chia and hemp-seeds; nuts and seeds like sunflower seeds, sesame seed, pecans, and walnut; avocado and soy-beans (but choose only organic and non-GMO).

If you are getting eggs from good sources, they are also higher in Omega-3. What might surprise you is that Omega-3 fatty acids are also found in dark leafy greens and the cruciferous vegetables like broccoli and cauliflower.

A last note if you have been eating fat-free for a while: Fat is, of course, also a high-calorie food, but the calories in good fats aren't the kind to be afraid of. We gain fat from eating sugar, not fat.

The trick with fat is to strike a balance. Your goal is to have fat (mostly unsaturated) account for a maximum of 25–30% of your daily diet. Depending on health issues, you might need less. Try adding some good healthy fats to your daily meals, and if you're not always getting enough Omega-3, you can add a supplement. But remember to think food first, since that's how you will master your appetite—a supplement can't do that for you. Once you start feeling more satiated from your food, you'll also learn how to stop eating when you're full. Learn to read the signs of hunger, and trust your body—it knows what it needs!

In a nutshell, here are my guidelines for choosing healthy fats:

- Get most of your fat from plant foods such as avocado, nuts, seeds, and healthy oils.

- Limit animal fat from meat and dairy; choose plant-fats and fish instead.

- Get a high-quality Omega-3 supply every day from chia, flax or hemp seeds; flaxseed or hempseed oil; dark leafy greens and other vegetables; fish; or eggs high in Omega-3. You can also add a good fish oil supplement if needed.

- For cooking, choose the right oil for your cooking temperature according to the guidelines laid out above and what the oil states on its label. Avoid any oil that comes from a genetically modified source.

FRUIT: THE SWEET NECTAR OF NATURE

How much fruit is enough?
Naturally sweet fruit is an important alternative to candy bars and other sugary foods, but we do have to be mindful of the fact that fruit is high in

fructose (natural sugar). Fruit can help you beat your cravings, but it isn't as good at helping you master your appetite as vegetables, with their high fiber and low glycemic index. This doesn't mean that fruit is "bad" for you—it means you'll want to think of fruit in proportion to your other choices. One or two servings per day is enough. It's a great snack, but it's not a great meal.

Why local and seasonal is best

When choosing what fruit to eat, think of the season you're in and consider what's grown in your part of the country. Fresh, locally grown fruits are always the healthiest choice, in part because fruit affects your body temperature—for example, a tropical fruit consumed in the middle of an East Coast winter is going to have a cooling effect just when you don't need it. Your satisfaction from eating locally grown fruit is also higher because food that has traveled less was likely picked when it was riper, which means it had time to develop more micronutrients. Remember that the more nutrients your body absorbs, the more satisfied you'll feel after eating (and the less likely you'll be to overeat). Quality over quantity is the general rule. It might go without saying that canned fruit is much less nutritious than fresh, and it's often packed in sugar-syrup to boot! Also, many conventionally grown fruits are sprayed with pesticides and are better eaten sparingly or avoided altogether: Always choose organic or low-spray when possible, and wash any non-organic fruit well before eating.

Fruit, energy levels, and digestion

The sweetness of fruit can provide a surge of energy just when we need it. A little fruit can be delicious cooked in with savory dishes, but be aware that for some people the combination of fruit with foods other than greens can lead to poor digestion, bloating and discomfort—which will in turn lead to feeling less satisfied from a meal. Experiment, and see how different combinations affect you.

Fruit is a healthy choice for dessert in the place of something sugary, but it's always best to give yourself some time to digest your meal first for the reason mentioned above. Also, remember that it takes about twenty minutes for your stomach to tell your brain how full you actually are, so I suggest waiting a full twenty minutes before reaching for that apple or pear—and always drink a glass of water after the meal and before considering whether you're hungry for dessert. Sometimes all you'll need is a naturally sweet tea, which will soothe a sugar craving and also aid in digestion. Licorice, mint, ginger, and other herbal teas are nice after-meal drinks.

To juice or not to juice?

Juices and smoothies are popularly seen as healthy drink choices, but while they are healthier than soda, they still pack a high sugar content; the sugar in fruit (fructose) is natural, but it can still spike your blood-glucose levels, causing you to get false hunger cravings. There's also the question of portion size: Think of how many pieces of fruit go into a single smoothie or a single glass of juice compared to how many pieces you'd be likely to eat as a snack.

Fruit juices are less desirable because the juicing process removes all of the fiber from a fruit, significantly reducing the benefits of eating the fruit whole, and also causing a faster absorption of sugar into the bloodstream. If you really want to drink your fruit, I suggest making smoothies that contain a lot of vegetables (particularly leafy greens) along with some fat like avocado, and adding just a small amount of fruit for sweetness and flavor.

Fruit and your overall health: The mighty antioxidant

Fruit is high in phytochemicals and antioxidants, so it's a nice added daily dose of health (of course, vegetables are high in these nutrients too). Antioxidants are naturally occurring plant substances that block and protect your cells from free radicals, which cause the oxidation of cells— similar to rust on a car. Our cell health is being destroyed by the rise of free radicals in our environment from pollution, over-processed foods, and additives. The resulting cell damage can lead to premature aging (including your skin!), heart disease, cancer, and a general weakening of the immune system. Some antioxidants block free radicals, others make them less damaging, and some even repair the cells that are damaged. Antioxidants include vitamin C, vitamin E, and beta carotene, which is converted to vitamin A in the body as it is needed. Fruits high in antioxidants include tart cherries, wild blueberries and other berries, watermelon and melons in general, and apples. Interestingly, beans top the charts in antioxidants, along with other vegetables you might not expect, like fennel.

Fruit and appetite

As with all food groups, fruits vary in nutritional value. Some are high in vitamins, some in fiber, some in sugar (fructose). If you're in need of a quick energy boost and pick-me-up in place of a candy bar, dried fruit gives you the fastest release of sugar into the bloodstream. Fresh fruit gives you a slower release of sugar, which translates to more stable, longer lasting energy. *But keep in mind that fructose has also been shown in studies to increase appetite*. Vegetables are often a better choice: a carrot is sweet but packed with fiber, making it even more sustainable as an energy source and a way of mastering your appetite.

You'll get more appetite-mastering benefit from fruit if you top it with a little nut butter (apples and almond butter make a great combination). The fat and protein in the nut butter prolongs a feeling of satiety by slowing down both the absorption and the release of the sugars from the apple. Whatever prolongs the absorption and release of sugar contributes to a steady energy level, which in turn reduces the chance that a sugar craving will hit.

We tend to under-eat and over-snack, so when you are considering snacking on fruit, remember: Less is better!

→ When it comes to fruit, quality over quantity is the general rule.

→ Smoothies and juices contain much more fruit than you would be likely to eat as a snack.

→ Sometimes all you'll need for dessert is a naturally sweet tea, which will soothe a sugar craving and also aid in digestion.

VITAMINS & MINERALS

The essentials

Our food is not just carbohydrates, protein, and fat. Our food is our supply of vitamins and minerals, which you can think of as the building blocks of our blood and of every single cell in our bodies. Vitamins and minerals are crucial not only for our general health but also, as we've learned, for mastering our appetite, cravings, and mood because we need to absorb a certain amount of nutrients, vitamins, and minerals to feel satisfied.

This means that when you're truly satisfied by your food, your entire body—not just your stomach but also your organs and cells—is being fed with the nurture that it needs.

The source of this nurture is our food—especially when it is high quality, cooked well (not over-cooked), locally sourced and fresh. Unfortunately, many of our foods are mass-produced, grown in unfavorable conditions, and/or imported from far away (and therefore harvested before getting the chance to mature and develop the right nutrient levels). You can think of it this way: The better quality you choose, the better you will feel. If we can't get all of our nutrients from food, we might sometimes need to add supplements. But we cannot completely replace our healthy foods with pills; those who believe that if they take the right supplements their food choices don't matter are not clear on the true meaning of nourishment, and they lose out on feeling satiated too. Supplements are supplements—not a replacement for real, yummy food.

Fortunately, nature has already designed most of its food to contain a variety of nutrients, vitamins, and minerals that mutually support each other and assist in the absorption and assimilation of this bounty. *This is why a varied and balanced selection of good food choices is more vital that your multivitamin.*

Fat- and water-soluble vitamins

One of the reasons fats are important in your daily diet is because certain vitamins are only absorbed when ingested with fats. These fat-soluble vitamins are stored in your body and released over time, so you can actually get too much of them if you add them as supplements. They include vitamin A, vitamin D, vitamin E, and vitamin K.

Water-soluble vitamins are not stored in your body and in fact are lost when you urinate, so you need a more consistent supply of them. These easy-come, easy-go vitamins are fuel for the body's metabolism, digestive system, cells, blood, and organs. They're found in fruit, vegetables, and grains. Because these vitamins are destroyed by heat and excess air, we want to consume the foods that contain them as fresh as possible, and closer to raw than to overcooked—steaming and sautéing vegetables preserves their vitamins better than boiling, for example. Again, local is better, since long transport times can lead to increased exposure to heat and air. The water-soluble vitamins include: vitamin B12, vitamin C, biotin, folic acid, niacin, pantothenic acid, riboflavin, and thiamin.

Vitamin D: The one supplement you may need to take

I remember my mother giving me cod-liver oil as a child for its vitamin D and Omega-3 fatty acids. Even though we ate a lot of fish, we had so little sunshine (the main source of vitamin D) during Denmark's long winters that our vitamin D levels could get too low. Today, even in countries that aren't as northern as Denmark, we tend not to get enough sunshine because we work inside. As a result, many of us will need to supplement our vitamin D intake. Choose a good quality supplement rather than fortified foods (like orange juice with added vitamin D), since fortification is a form of the processing we are trying in general to avoid.

Vitamin D is beneficial in a number of different ways. It's necessary for the absorption of calcium and therefore adds to bone strength; calcium deficiency has also been shown to be a factor in insulin resistance and obesity. Since calcium supplements interfere with chromium (which is essential for mastering your appetite and cravings), it's better to take a vitamin D supplement and get your calcium naturally from food—leafy greens, nuts, seeds, and wild salmon are good sources, and for the reasons I outlined in the chapter on dairy I recommend them all over milk.

This vitamin is also important for the functioning of about 200 genes in our system and has been found to be a key player in cancer prevention, as well as in mood and brain function. And lack of the "sunshine vitamin" has been shown to correlate to Seasonal Affective Disorder (SAD), also known as the "winter blues." (But remember that food choices can also affect mood, and sugar in particular can lead to mood instability, while vitamin D and Omega-3 fatty acids can help battle depression.)

As if that isn't enough, Vitamin D also helps regulate the immune system and prevent inflammation. This makes it particularly important for autoimmune diseases such as diabetes, rheumatoid arthritis, MS, and IBS. Lastly, vitamin D is essential for thyroid functions, which influence our metabolisms. This is important for weight management and for health in general and helps explain why a lack of vitamin D can show up as fatigue and even depression. One fact that isn't widely known yet is that vitamin D also has an effect on blood-sugar control and insulin resistance. This is another reason it might be crucial for mastering your appetite and cravings.

Vitamin D is one of the fat-soluble vitamins, which means if we don't include dietary fat—like the Omega-3 fatty acids—in our choices, we don't absorb this vitamin well. It also means that if we're carrying too much body fat, vitamin D can get absorbed into those fat cells and remain stored there, making it less available in our blood where we need it.

Minerals: The micro world of nurture

Minerals are as important as vitamins, and they are also essential for the absorption of vitamins. While the body can produce some vitamins by itself, it cannot produce minerals.

Minerals are found in a variety of foods such as wholegrain, cereals, vegetables, fresh and dried fruit, nuts and seeds, and fish; they are also in dairy and meat products (though I don't recommend eating a lot of those foods). They are fundamental for major functions of your body such as building bones and teeth, soft tissue, muscles, blood, and nerve cells; controlling the fluids in the body and cells; and converting food into usable energy. Minerals are also crucial for general mental and physical health.

The essential minerals are: calcium, iron, magnesium, phosphorus, potassium, sodium, and sulfur. Trace minerals are indispensable but needed in much smaller amounts than other vitamins and minerals. They are necessary to protect cells and nerves, and for metabolizing energy; they support digestion, hormone balance, and enzymes, and they're also required for the assimilation of other vitamins and minerals. Just like minerals, trace minerals—which include boron, cobalt, copper, chromium, fluoride, iodine, manganese, molybdenum, selenium, silicon, and zinc—are found in a variety of foods. But they are often lacking in our food sources today because of depleted soil and because we often don't eat enough locally sourced foods. Your farmers' markets are the best option for sourcing foods richer with trace minerals.

Two special cases: Chromium and Magnesium
Chromium, a trace mineral, is a very important factor in blood-sugar regulation and therefore in mastering your appetite. In fact, chromium plays a fundamental role in glucose tolerance, insulin, and the metabolism of cholesterol. When we eat

a meal, our insulin levels go up in response to the glucose we take in. Chromium is essential to balancing the glucose that enters our cells.

If we are deficient in chromium, we can become resistant to insulin. There is an indication that many people in the United States are deficient partly because they eat too much processed food, from which the natural chromium has been removed. Chromium is also essential for rebuilding damaged DNA in our cells, and it can affect our mood as well. This may be related to the fact that chromium helps balance our blood-sugar levels; stability in these levels correlates with a better mood, which also helps us master our appetites and cravings.

In addition to not getting enough chromium because of our food sources and choices, we also lose chromium due to stress, both physical and emotional. That's because when the levels of the stress hormone, cortisol, increase in the body, blood-sugar imbalances result, causing a greater need for and use of chromium. We also excrete more chromium through our urine when we are eating a lot of simple sugars—another reason to get your sweetness from complex sources like wholegrain, root vegetables, and cooked onion, which are also some of the foods that provide chromium.

Magnesium helps in the absorption of fats, protein, and carbohydrates, and of the nutrients they contain. This is, as you have learned, an essential factor in being satiated from your meals so you can avoid overeating. It also assists in balancing insulin and in the metabolism of glucose—also important for mastering your appetite. When you are low in magnesium, you can feel fatigued, and then you might also crave more sugar to give you energy.

Magnesium is found in leafy greens and green vegetables, nuts and seeds, avocado, fish (including mackerel, wild salmon and halibut), bananas, and very dark chocolate (to get health benefits from chocolate, choose 80% or darker, without dairy or processed sugar added).

> → Supplements are supplements—not a replacement for real yummy food.

> → Vitamin D is one vitamin you may need to get from a good-quality supplement (preferred over fortified foods, such as orange juice with added vitamin D).

→ While the body can produce many vitamins on its own, it cannot produce minerals. Your farmers' markets are the best option for sourcing foods that are fresher, therefore richer with trace minerals.

→ Natural sources of chromium include whole-grain, root vegetables and onion; magnesium is found in leafy greens and green vegetables, nuts and seeds, avocado, some types of fish, bananas, and very dark chocolate.

HEALTH BY COLOR

One way to make sure you get the nutrients you need in a meal is to notice the colors of the food you eat. The pigmentation that gives each fruit and vegetable its color is directly related to its nutritional value; once you learn some rules of thumb, getting the variety you need becomes easy and fun. In traditional Chinese medicine, each color of food also represents specific organs; eating food of that color nourishes and balances those organs. The Chinese system also connects specific emotions to each organ, emphasizing how food nourishes more than just the stomach. So: Color up your plate. Here's how.

Green

In short, go green! It's a very easy way to add healthy choices to each meal. Because of their "superfood" health benefits, greens are an exception to my general advice to eat only locally when possible: Good greens are now widely available year round wherever you are, and it's worth finding greens even out of season. A great source of vitamins (including folate, one of the B vitamins) as well as minerals and fiber, greens get their color from chlorophyll. Kale, collard greens, broccoli, peas, and field greens like arugula also contain the all-important antioxidants known as carotenoids (more on those below). Cruciferous vegetables such as cabbage, Brussels sprouts, cauliflower (though not green), and kale contain not only antioxidants and other phytonutrients but also indoles that reduce cancer risk by blocking carcinogens from reaching the cells; indoles protect against DNA damage, too, and assist in converting damaging estrogen to safe estrogen.

All the leafy greens, especially dark ones, are particularly powerful choices: kale, collards, bok choy, endives, mustard greens, Swiss chard, field greens, mesclun salad, arugula, watercress, and spinach (my least favorite because of the high acid levels). For non-leafy vegetables, choose artichokes, asparagus, broccoli, broccoli rabe, Brussels sprouts, Chinese cabbage, green beans, green cabbage, celery, peas, and sugar snap peas. For extra green super-power, try the green powdered drinks (mixed with water) made from cereal grasses such as wheat grass and barley grass. Popeye watch out!

For fruit, try green apples, green grapes, kiwi, lime, and green pears.

In Chinese medicine, green foods—especially bitter greens—are connected to the liver and the gallbladder, organs that hold the emotions of anger and will.

Orange/Yellow

The pigment that colors orange and yellow fruits and vegetables comes from the group of antioxidants known as carotenoids. Rich in beta carotene, these phytochemicals boost our immune systems and have been shown to protect our eyes against cataracts and macular degeneration; studies have also demonstrated a decrease in bad cholesterol with an increased intake of vegetables high in carotenoids. Orange fruits and vegetables also give you vitamin C and folate, which is needed to reduce the risk of heart disease and prevent certain birth defects. As an added benefit, many yellow- and orange-pigmented foods also contain bioflavonoids, which are believed to have beneficial anti-inflammatory properties.

Some good choices include: yellow beets, butternut squash, carrots, pumpkin, yams, and sweet potatoes.

For fruit: apricots, cantaloupe, grapefruit, lemon, mangoes, oranges, papayas, peaches, yellow apples and pears, persimmons.

Orange and yellow foods nourish the spleen and stomach and are connected to the emotions of worry and empathy. They add some of the sweetness we crave in our foods and help soothe our digestion, too.

Red
Red-pigmented fruits and vegetables contain lycopene. This is a powerful antioxidant that helps to fight heart disease and some types of cancer, particularly prostate cancer. It can also assist in increasing memory functions. For vegetables, try

beets, red beans, radicchio, red onions, and rhubarb. Tomatoes, red potatoes, and red peppers are also part of this group, but note that these are "nightshade" vegetables and not recommended for those with arthritis and osteoporosis. So called because they grow at night, nightshade vegetables contain high levels of alkaloids, which can cause bones to excrete calcium, other minerals, and trace elements from the body. They can affect nerve muscle functions and the digestive system and can cause inflammation in the joints. Eggplant, spinach, and tobacco are some of the other nightshade vegetables.

For fruit, choose red apples, blood oranges, cherries, cranberries, red grapes, pink/red grapefruit, red pears, pomegranates, raspberries, strawberries, and watermelon.

Red foods nourish and balance our hearts and small intestines; their emotions are joy and happiness as well as the opposite emotion of sadness.

Black, blue, and purple
Blue and purple fruits and vegetables may be your best defense against the effects of aging. The blue pigment in blueberries, purple grapes, red cabbage, beets, and plums comes from

anthocyaninsms, phytochemicals that protect cells against damage from carcinogens; they may also help prevent heart disease and improve memory function.

Be black and blue with: beans, seaweed, black sesame, black mushrooms, and purple cabbage.

For fruit: blackberries, blueberries, black currants, dried plums, purple figs, purple grapes, plums, and raisins.

Black foods are connected to the kidneys, which are related to fear and courage. Kidney stagnation is a common diagnosis; to prevent it, make sure not to eat too much salt, and drink plenty of water.

White, tan, and brown

Garlic and the onion family, as well as other white-hued vegetables, are colored with anthoxanthins and contain allicin, another phytochemical that may help lower both cholesterol levels and blood pressure. It may also assist in reducing the risk of stomach cancer.

Add these benefits to your plate with: cauliflower, daikon, garlic, ginger, Jerusalem artichoke, jicama, mushrooms, onions, parsnips, radishes, shallots, turnips, leeks, scallions, and white fish. For fruit: bananas, brown pears, dates, and prunes.

White represents the lungs and is connected to the emotions of grief and loss.

→ In traditional Chinese medicine, each color of food also represents specific organs; eating food of that color nourishes and balances those organs.

→ Go green! It's a very easy way to add healthy choices to each meal.

SUPERFOODS FOR MASTERING APPETITE

Everybody is talking about Superfoods—it's been a buzzword for years, and it isn't going anywhere. Here are some reasons why:

- Superfoods are high in fiber, vitamins, minerals, and other nutrients.

- They're high in phytonutrients and antioxidant compounds, such as vitamins A, E, and beta carotene.

- They contribute to reducing the risk of heart disease and other health conditions by preventing and reducing inflammation.

- They can help protect against cancer.

- They help to promote digestive health.

- They help protect cells and eliminate toxins.

That all adds up to you feeling better, healthier, and more satisfied from your food.

There are many Superfoods, but here are the top ten—all of them familiar foods that are easy to add to your daily meals:

Broccoli and the cruciferous family
Besides being a good source of calcium, potassium, folate, and fiber, broccoli also contains high levels of phytonutrients that can help prevent heart disease, diabetes, and some cancers. Broccoli is also a good source of vitamins A and C, which protect your body's cells from damage. The fiber content and nutrient density of cruciferous vegetables make them an excellent choice both for improving your health and for mastering your appetite.

Beans and lentils

Beans—especially red beans, including adzuki, anasazi, and kidney beans, as well as lentils—are good sources of iron, magnesium, phosphorus, potassium, copper, and thiamin. Red beans also contain the phytonutrients that can help prevent cardiovascular disease and cancer. All legumes—including black and white beans, peas, and lentils—are excellent low-calorie sources of plant protein and dietary fiber, which makes them powerful aids to mastering your appetite and promoting overall health.

Dark leafy greens

Dark leafy greens such as arugula, kale, collard greens, spinach, and sprouts are high in vitamins A and C and folate and are also a good source of riboflavin, vitamin B-6, calcium, iron, and magnesium. The plant nutrients in leafy greens and sprouts help support the detoxification functions of the liver, cleanse the intestines, and boost your immune system. The darker the leafy greens, the denser their fiber structure—and the more satisfying. Low in calories and starch and high in fiber and nutrient levels, dark leafy greens are great for mastering your weight and appetite. (Once again, a note that spinach is in the nightshade family.)

Sweet potatoes and yams

The deep orange-yellow color of sweet potatoes tells you they are high in the antioxidant beta carotene. Food sources of beta carotene, which gets converted to vitamin A in your body, can help to slow the aging process and reduce the risk of some cancers. Sweet potatoes are also a good source of fiber; vitamins B-6, C and E; folate; and potassium. Like all vegetables, they are relatively low in sugar and calories, and high in nutrients—in other words, fantastic for mastering your appetite. Furthermore, the sweetness they add to a meal helps you feel satisfied and can prevent a sweet-tooth snack attack later on.

Nuts and seeds

Nuts offer myriad health benefits. Common nuts like walnuts, almonds, pecans, and pistachios are packed with nutrients—fiber, Omega-3 fatty acids, riboflavin, magnesium, iron, and calcium. Specific benefits vary, of course: Almonds, for example, are especially high in calcium and provide a good source of vitamin E. Nuts are also an excellent plant source of protein, and they're good for your heart because of their monounsaturated fat, the healthier type of fat that can help lower cholesterol. And don't forget seeds like pumpkin, sunflower, and sesame, which are also high in nutrients, Omega-3 fatty acids, and fiber, as well as protein. They're all great choices for topping a salad or munching on as a snack.

Wholegrain

As we learned in the chapter on wholegrain, these grassy plants (when consumed unprocessed and unrefined) are good sources of complex carbohydrates and various vitamins and minerals. Wholegrain helps to stabilize blood sugar and insulin and can protect against heart disease. Among many health benefits from complex carbohydrates, grains high in fiber help detoxify the intestines. A high-fiber diet also makes a meal more satisfying and keeps you feeling full longer, making wholegrain crucial for mastering your appetite and cravings.

Wild salmon

Salmon is high in protein, low in saturated fat and cholesterol, and rich in calcium, selenium, vitamin D, and vitamin E. It is one of the best sources of Omega-3 fatty acids—the "good fat" that has so many health benefits, including fighting depression, increasing cognitive ability, and helping to prevent the formation of blood clots that may cause heart attacks. It can also help decrease triglyceride levels and the growth of artery-clogging plaques, while lowering blood pressure and thereby reducing the risk of stroke. Providing both a complete protein and all the benefits of healthy fats, wild salmon is an excellent choice for optimum mastery of your appetite and your health—but do note that farmed salmon does not have the same benefits; consider the source of any farmed fish you eat, choosing sustainable farms that avoid the use of antibiotics.

Other good fish choices include cod, halibut, haddock, monkfish, mackerel, herring, eel, and plaice (flatfish, like sole and flounder). Tuna is not a sure choice these days because of higher levels of mercury and toxins (bigger fish, more toxins), so it's better to consume it in moderation. Because of distinctions in water quality and fishing practices, toxicity levels in fish vary greatly; if you want to make fish a significant part of your diet, it's best to consult the resources available online at seafoodwatch.org. You will also add to global health by making sure you choose more eco-sustainable sources of fish, since the fishing industry is not always a healthy one.

Apples

Apples contain pectin, a soluble fiber that can lower blood cholesterol and glucose levels. Fresh apples are also good sources of vitamin C, which protects cells and contributes to the production of collagen, the connective tissue that keeps your capillaries and blood vessels healthy. Apples also support the absorption of iron and folate. Due to their high fiber and relatively low glycemic index, apples are one source of sweetness that will help keep your blood-sugar levels steady. Remember that both fiber and blood-sugar balance are essential for mastering your appetite and your cravings.

Berries

Blueberries, especially the wild kind, are a rich source of plant compounds called phytonutrients. The specific phytonutrients in blueberries are believed to promote healthy aging and help improve short-term memory. Both cranberries and blueberries can prevent urinary tract infections. Blueberries are more of a savory berry, high in nutrients, especially vitamin C and beta-carotene, and rich in fiber. This makes them a better berry choice for mastering your cravings.

Liquid superfoods: What to drink

Your best choices are pure spring or purified water and green tea. Many think of coffee as a way to suppress appetite, but we all know from experience that this effect is only temporary. Also, the way coffee temporarily suppresses appetite is by heightening your stress levels! Coffee affects the adrenal glands, which produce the stress hormone cortisol. Because a release of stress hormones is always followed by a dip in energy levels, drinking coffee sets you onto a dangerous cycle: After your first fix, your sugar cravings and hunger signals will increase, making you crave sugar, starch—or more coffee, which leads to more cravings, until eventually you will probably give in.

Water is the best drink for mastering your appetite and your cravings. Drinking a large glass of fresh and pure water several times throughout the day ensures you won't get dehydrated, a feeling that is often confused with hunger and fatigue—all of which can easily lead to sugar cravings. Drinking enough water is simply essential for health and well-being. The general daily recommendation is to drink one-half of your body weight in ounces. That is one of the easiest ways to keep your body feeling optimal, along with the next best choice for drinking: green tea.

Along with its metabolism-boosting effects, green tea has high levels of an antioxidant compound called ECGC that can, according to several studies, protect against cancer. It helps trigger the reset button in immune systems that have been weakened by high insulin levels—another cancer-fighting benefit. By keeping both insulin and blood-sugar levels low and steady, green tea is also a great craving-buster—much preferred to coffee or soda, both of which increase glucose levels and trigger hunger. But be aware that drinking too much of it may cause increased stomach acidity in some people, so you need to find what works for you. And don't drink it on an empty stomach or you might get nauseous.

The chocolate fantasy

For many people, chocolate is a favorite treat. Why is that? The answer is simple: It makes us feel good. Another very soulful and nourishing reason for craving chocolate lies beyond the obvious one.

Chocolate affects our mood hormones: serotonin, endorphins, and phenylethylamine. Serotonin is our antidepressant hormone. It makes us feel good, emotionally stable, and calm. Endorphins are also released during exercise—they make us feel enthusiastic and powerful. Phenylethylamine is the very same hormone our body releases in response to love.

The taste of chocolate is, of course, its greatest allure; but it also satisfies our cravings for fat and carbohydrates. One of the reasons women tend to crave chocolate around the time of their period is that the change in estrogen levels can make us crave more fat and carbs. It's the body's instinctive response to the possibility of pregnancy, in which case the fetus would need the added nutritional energy. But as we have learned, what the body really wants in the way of energy is good complex carbohydrates, so going for sugar is not the answer.

The important thing to remember about chocolate is that there is a vast difference between the nutritional values of a candy bar from the supermarket and a bar of high-quality, very dark (80% or darker) chocolate containing almost no sugar or dairy.

Commercial chocolate bars contain so many other things besides chocolate that they almost always fall into the category of junk food and are best avoided.

The benefits that are found in raw and very dark chocolate come from the nutrients found in raw cacao: essential minerals such as potassium, magnesium, copper, potassium; polyphenols (which are believed to act as antioxidants), and vitamins including B1, B2, D, and E. The naturally occurring fat in chocolate is cocoa butter, which contains both monounsaturated and saturated fat (primarily stearic acid)—but like coconut oil, it's an exception to the general rule and does not raise bad cholesterol levels. Add to that the presence in stearic acid of flavonoids, which neutralize free radicals and are known to improve blood-vessel flexibility, and it's easy to see why dark chocolate is often promoted as a Superfood.

A small amount of dark chocolate is a nice way to give your Self a treat after a healthy meal. The higher fat in dark chocolate can help satiate you more than lighter chocolate, which can trigger a desire to keep eating; lighter chocolate contains more refined sugar and dairy, so it can easily take you to the trance-like state of the "bliss-point," where you feel out of control. Lighter chocolate is also not a healthy treat because the sugar and dairy cancel out the benefits of the antioxidants in the chocolate itself—dairy actually interferes with the absorption of flavonoids, for example.

But there are reasons to be mindful of your intake of even the darkest chocolate: For many of us, chocolate is a trigger food that can easily lead to an all-out binge. Because of our emotional relationship with treats, and because of how chocolate affects the hormones that make us feel loved, in darker moments we can be inclined to bury ourselves in a chocolate indulgence. This is especially dangerous for people with diabetes. While dark chocolate can often be safe for them to eat in small quantities, in excess it can act like any other candy bar and other sweets that wreak havoc on their insulin levels.

The bottom line: Think of chocolate as a treat, not a food. Eat dark chocolate only in small amounts, and don't depend on it for your antioxidants and flavonoids—as we have learned, these can all be found in vegetables, fruits, and green tea, all of which are much more powerful tools for reaching your goals of health, appetite mastery, and real satisfaction.

→ Legumes—including black and white beans, peas, and lentils are excellent high-nutrient, low-calorie sources of plant protein and dietary fiber, which makes them powerful aids to mastering your appetite and promoting overall health.

→ Low in calories and starch and high in fiber and nutrient levels, dark leafy greens are great for mastering your weight and appetite.

→ The sweetness in sweet potatoes and yams helps you to feel satisfied and can prevent a sweet-tooth snack attack after a meal.

→ Coffee affects the adrenal glands, which produces the stress hormone cortisol. Instead, drink more water to master your appetite and your cravings: 1/2 your body weight in ounces each day.

→ Green tea is also a great craving-buster—much preferred to coffee or soda, both of which increase glucose levels and trigger hunger.

→ Try filling and nutritious nuts and seeds as a topper for a salad or as a healthy snack.

→ Check seafoodwatch.org for updated information on the health value (and possible contamination) of the fish you eat.

→ Very dark chocolate has health benefits, but think of it as a treat, not a food.

REAL FOOD FOR THE REAL YOU

Pretty much everything we've discussed so far has centered around one fundamental question: What choices can you make so that you will get everything you need—sustenance, health, pleasure, weight loss, and a feeling of satiety—from the food on your plate?

Let's pause to revisit the way this book began. Say the word "food": What comes to mind now? See if what you imagine on your plate has changed after what you've learned so far.

Now, let's consider some of the questions that have come up in passing as we discussed various foods and their benefits. Do you want to eat whole foods or refined foods? Real foods or processed foods? Where does your food come from—who grew it or raised it, and how did it get to your kitchen? And the big question: Are convenience and the temporary high of junk food really more valuable than the health of you and your family, not to mention the health of the planet?

Your answer to that last question is probably "of course not!" But we all know how easy it is to succumb to convenience and the quick-fix of an unhealthy processed snack. So let's take a moment to revisit the importance of eating real food—for the real you.

Processing and refining

You know by now that the more you eat food in its original context, the more nutrients your body will absorb. In turn, you'll become better nourished and healthier, and you'll feel more whole and satisfied from the food you eat. When you connect more with your food, you connect more with your Self.

A whole food is a food that has had none of its components removed. To take the example of wheat, this would be the whole wheat berry. A *processed* food is one that has undergone some kind of transformation—cooking, grinding, pureeing, drying—so whole wheat flour, which is ground but has had no part of the berry removed, is essentially a processed food. A *refined* food is one that has been stripped of some of its inherent components, often the part with the fiber in it; the refined version of wheat would be white flour, in which the wheat germ and bran have been removed before grinding. Not all processed foods are "bad" for you—cooking (not overcooking) is a basic process that can enhance the flavor and digestibility of vegetables while retaining most of their nutritional value. And carrot juice, for example, is both processed (juiced) and refined (the fiber is removed), but it still has lots of vitamins, and though I don't recommend overdoing it, it's certainly healthier than soda!

Highly processed and highly refined foods—like those in fast food and packaged food—are what you want to avoid as much as possible. Refining depletes the nutrition from a naturally healthy food, but nutrition is also lost when we add unhealthy ingredients to a natural food—so we want to avoid canned vegetables (which often have sugar added), for example, or packaged cold cuts that contain nitrates and no longer even remotely resemble the animals from which they came. And remember what we've learned so far: When it comes to mastering your appetite, it's the fiber in whole foods that makes a meal the most sustaining. Once your body has learned this, you'll find yourself instinctively reaching for whole instead of processed and refined foods.

Food processing (which includes fermenting) goes back literally for centuries, and certain kinds of refining are very traditional practices too. But the beginning of our modern era of over-processed and packaged-for-convenience foods can be traced to the single ingredient that is present in almost all packaged and fast food: refined sugar.

Sugar

People originally chewed sugarcane (a whole food, packed with fiber) to extract the sweetness from it. Around 350 A.D., Indians discovered how to crystallize sugar, and later it became a trade commodity. It took centuries before the process was optimized and the international market was tapped; in the seventeenth and eighteenth centuries, sugar was traded in the Western world as if it were gold. For the aristocrats of France and England with a sweet tooth, the more refined the sugar was, the fancier it seemed. But then strange illnesses started to emerge, illnesses that seemed to relate to malnutrition, which was confusing to the otherwise well-fed wealthy class. Interestingly enough, the slaves who chewed on sugarcane while harvesting it (but who weren't offered the sweets made from refined sugar that their masters consumed) didn't end up suffering the same illnesses as did the upper classes. We now know the reason: The refining process had removed the fiber and nutrients from the sugarcane, resulting in a nutritionally "empty" food!

Refined sugar isn't just empty, it's actively unhealthy for our triglyceride and cholesterol levels, and as you already know, it increases the risk of diabetes. What you may not know is that it also depletes and weakens your immune system and increases mucus in your body, causing respiratory congestion, an overgrowth of bacteria in your intestinal system, and the production of phlegm. The more refined sugar you get from your food and prepared meals, the more your blood-sugar levels will become imbalanced, leading to excessive hunger and food cravings; sugar also behaves like an addictive substance, and it can take very little of it to trigger a binge.

We have to be more careful now than ever about accidentally consuming sugar. In its early heyday, sugar was expensive so it was consumed in much smaller quantities then than it is now, when it's present in everything from the obvious—candies, cookies, and cakes—to the less obvious, such as canned and packaged foods, salad dressings, sauces, even French fries. Added sugar in foods can be a surprise discovery because we don't expect it where we think it's not needed. It's used in marinated, pickled, and preserved foods. It's used to extend the shelf life of packaged foods and to make fat-free foods taste better. From ketchup to salad dressings to smoked salmon, added sugar is everywhere in the grocery aisles. And by now we know very well that while adding sugar to food might make it taste better, it also has a tendency to make us overeat and get stuck in the cycle of hunger and cravings that is so hard to break.

The packaged and fast-food industries know very well that sugary foods will make you want to eat—and buy—more; and as if that's not enough, they have discovered the perfect combination of sugar, fat, and salt to create a "bliss-point" that is so addictive it's almost impossible to resist. This bliss-point is a physical reality, affecting the brain's addiction center in such a way that you'll feel like you're in a trance once you start eating the food. And you are.

Tips and tricks for staying real

It's not easy to avoid something as ubiquitous as sugar—or the trio of sugar-fat-salt that food processors are banking on. Here are some tips and tricks for staying real.

- Avoid packaged, refined, and unnecessarily processed foods as much as possible.

- If you eat packaged food, read the labels and avoid any containing trans fat, any products labeled "fat-free," and anything with an excess amount of sugar.

- Whenever you eat sugar, add healthy fats to your meal; this will slow down the absorption of the sugar into your bloodstream.

- Remember that it's about proportion, not portion. Think about *balancing* your meals.

- Cook at home as much as you can, using fresh produce and processing it as little as possible while retaining taste and nourishment.

- When you eat out, look for restaurants that mention the source of their food on their menus; these tend to be the businesses that are giving thought to the health of their customers, not only to their bottom line.

- Remember that the more whole foods you eat, the more you are benefiting not only your own health but that of the planet, since processing, refining, and packaging use energy from fossil fuels and create waste, and factory farming produces more greenhouse gases.

If you want to learn more ways to understand and master your food cravings, consider signing up for my online program, which provides even more insight into the relationship between food, nourishment, and thriving.

THE BALANCED MEAL: PUTTING IT ALL TOGETHER

Balance means different things to different people; it also varies depending on circumstances, time of day, and so on. The important thing to realize is that you are the only one who can find your own balance with respect to your eating habits and food choices. Not an easy task—but I'll give you some guidelines to work with.

Balance is also not a goal in and of itself; it's something that's constantly shifting. And that's the whole point of balance—it's always in flux. Balance is what we do to live in health: the actions we take, the choices we make, the thoughts we have, and the perspectives we hold.

This means that before each meal, you'll want to slow down for a moment to make note of your energy level, hunger, mood, the time of day, what activities you still need or want to engage in, and so on. Remember, you are the one who will know best what you need. This does ask of you that you be involved in your own care. Taking responsibility for our choices is often something we have a hard time with, and in the beginning we want someone else to tell us what to do. But once we own our choices, we feel empowered and we can keep improving our habits of self-care and our health. The more you learn about your Self, the more mindful you become about your patterns, choices, and emotions, and the more you learn how to change your habits, the more you will live the life you want.

These topics are too large for the scope of this book but they are among the primary focuses of the Path for Life online program.

For now, we will concentrate on some simple food-knowledge guidelines for creating a balanced meal that will satisfy your hunger and help you master your appetite and your cravings.

A meal for optimal satiation needs to be composed of certain elements. The combination of sweet, salt, and fat is something that is important to making us feel stimulated taste-wise, which is how the food industry came to discover the "bliss-point." But we want to learn how to feel that satiation and satisfaction without going into the trance-like state of wanting more—a state in which we find it hard to stop eating because it tastes *so good*. Now's a good time to slow down and just reflect on what I'm saying here: We want the "bliss" of tasty flavor, but we also want to avoid the trance so that we can recognize when we are satiated and feeling complete.

These general guidelines are simple to follow:

You need a balance of complex carbohydrates, both from vegetables and wholegrain; lean protein;

and healthy fats. Aim to satisfy your desire for all the different basic flavor sensations: sweet, bitter, sour, salty, and savory.

The proportions I suggest for a healthy plate are:

- ½ of your plate consists of yummy vegetables, preferably from the list of Superfoods that are so high in nutrients and fiber: a large proportion of leafy greens and other low-starch and cruciferous choices.

- ¼ of your plate consists of a cooked wholegrain and/or root vegetables.

- ¼ of your plate is taken up by lean protein, preferably from fish or legumes.

Make sure to cook with a *dash* of sea-salt to bring the taste out in the food, but avoid salting extra at the table without first tasting your food. In addition, I like to top off my vegetables with a good olive oil, maybe even mixed with lemon and herbs, for that extra serving of Omega-3 fatty acids and satisfying taste.

For your shopping list and some tips on cooking (the) basics, see the back of the book.

→ The food industry has invested heavily in discovering the "bliss point"—a combination of sweet, salt, and fat that triggers the brain's addiction center and effectively puts you in a trance. Seek true bliss from balanced meals made from whole foods instead.

→ Balance is not a goal in and of itself; it's something that's constantly shifting. Slow down before a meal and take note of your mood and hunger level.

HYDRATION

Our bodies are mostly water. Hydration is therefore an essential element of nurture for our entire system: organs, cells, tissue, and energy levels. So, for your health and well-being, you do want to drink plenty of fresh pure water.

But there's another excellent reason to increase the amount of water you drink: It affects your sense of satiation and will help stave off cravings.

Here's why:

Most people wait to drink water until they feel thirsty, which really means they're already dehydrated. Constant hunger and sweet cravings can very often be a sign of dehydration rather than of actual hunger. When they start drinking more water, many people find that they experience increased energy, better moods, less irritability, and more satiation over a longer period.

It's best to drink your water between meals; at mealtime, your body needs to focus on digesting food and absorbing and assimilating nutrients from it. We also can feel more bloated after a meal if we drink too much water with it. I suggest waiting twenty minutes after eating before drinking your water. This gives time for the food to settle in your stomach and begin to mix with the digestive enzymes. Since twenty minutes is also the amount of time it takes for the full satisfaction of a meal to sink in, this is also how long you will want to wait before deciding whether to have dessert. Water or a cup of tea might help you recognize the sensation of fullness, and you might very well find yourself passing on dessert—naturally.

There are many more reasons why we need water. Our digestive system requires water to function, especially when we eat foods high in fiber. Many people suffer from constipation because they don't drink enough water. Water is also essential to aid the body's natural detoxification system by flushing out toxins. Drinking water throughout the day or in larger quantities at different times in the day is also believed to help speed up your metabolism. You may not know that being hydrated is also important for our joints and muscles: Severe cramps, for example, can be a result of dehydration. Even backaches can be eased by drinking more water.

Some of the most typical symptoms of being low on water include headaches, fatigue, irritability, dry skin, false hunger, fuzziness, and difficulty focusing. It is believed that as many as 75% of Americans are chronically dehydrated. The normal recommendation is to drink a minimum of 8–10 eight-ounces glasses of water per day, but for many of us that might not even be enough, but since our needs vary according to our size, I recommend following the rule of thumb I mentioned before: Drink 50% of your body weight in ounces of water per day. But keep in mind that people with kidney issues may need either less or more water, and people who eat a lot of vegetables don't need as much water as meat eaters, since vegetables and wholegrain cooked in water also hydrate, while meat doesn't.

→ Water affects your sense of satiation and will help stave off cravings.

→ Drink your water between meals; at mealtime, your body needs to focus on digesting food and absorbing and assimilating nutrients from it.

→ Many people suffer from constipation because they don't drink enough water.

→ For maximum benefit, drink 50% of your body weight in ounces of water per day.

"Eat with all your senses, and you will feel so much more nourished."

HOW TO EAT

Feeling More Nourished From Your Food

GOOD EATING

Eat at the table

Yes, I mean at the table. It's essential to sit down at a table for a meal, or at least to sit down. Doing so on a park bench is certainly fine, too. But sitting is essential because it helps you take out a moment to be more mindful of the fact that you are eating.

Part of the point is to avoid multitasking while eating, so even if you're sitting down, it's not a good idea to try to read through email or work during your meal. Consider the fact that eating is an activity in itself. You may think that you can do more than one thing at a time and remain present to each thing. That's not the case. Your attention is a bit like a computer; it can be running several tasks in the background and have several windows open at the same time, but it can only actually focus on one of them at a time—you are the same way.

As difficult as it may be to just sit there and eat, try it. It will help you to master your appetite by being mindful of the act of eating and how you feel during it. I know that all the emotions come to the surface when you forgo distracting yourself with other things, but if it helps, just focus on the physical aspect of eating. That way, you can pay attention to the point at which you reach satisfaction from your food, and you can stop before you overeat. I know this is easier said than done, but don't give up. Give it a try, and keep practicing. You'll get better and better at it. Getting in touch with how your belly feels while you're eating is a whole new world for most people. But it is one of the keys to mindful eating, and mindful eating is the key to becoming more nourished and better able to master your appetite and your cravings. When you're stressed or struggling with emotional eating, this is particularly challenging. My next book will address more of these very essential—and actually very common—challenges to mindful eating.

Chewing

Mindful chewing is essential to feeling satiated and nourished, and it's one of the best defenses we have against overeating.

Pretty much everyone I know chews far less than is optimal except when they are truly paying attention to it. It's not easy to focus on chewing, or to learn to chew more; we don't have the habit, and it can feel awkward or cumbersome at first. I agree! But it is well worth it, and you'll get used to it in time.

Some say it's best to chew each bite 35–50 times. Short of having to sit there and count, you can make a simple rule for yourself: chew until the food is liquid in your mouth. Then swallow, and pay attention while you do so. The process of following your food mentally as it enters your body allows you to feel the sensation of the food filling up your stomach. If you do so, you'll notice that you reach a level of satiety long before you otherwise would have.

Chewing is crucial for your digestive health and for mastering your appetite. The grinding activity of our teeth and the enzymes in our saliva are essential to help us absorb the most nutrients from our food; together they begin to break food down in our mouths before it enters the stomach and the digestive tract. The digestion of carbohydrates starts in the mouth when they mix with saliva; that's one of the reasons you can feel bloated when you don't chew your food well.

The benefit of chewing for weight loss is twofold: You'll eat less food when you chew more because you absorb the nutrients better and feel more satiated; and chewing slows down your meal, helping you stop before overeating—as we know by now, it takes your brain twenty minutes to realize when you're full. The more you chew, the more you're giving your brain a chance to catch up with your mouth, and the more likely you are to realize you're full before your overeat. If you eat too fast, you end up eating an extra portion before realizing you're full—we've all been there. So basically, you'll feel more satiated from less food if you chew more. Simple and challenging—what a combination.

Frequency of eating

It is often recommended that we eat three meals per day and snacks in between. Some suggest five small meals per day instead. I tend to suggest the three real meals per day for most people. If we eat five small meals per day, it often turns into constant grazing. It can be hard to monitor your intake of food this way. A small meal often ends up becoming a bigger meal and, before we know it, we've had too much food for the day. Some end up under-eating at meals and over-snack for the rest of the day instead.

Our stomachs and digestive systems are set up to hold and process food without feeling hungry for a few hours in a row (3-4 hours, to be more precise). That's a good interval to let pass between meals.

Of course sometimes, your next meal will be more than five hours away—that's when a good snack comes in handy. But be careful about reaching for a snack automatically; you really only need a snack if you start feeling hungry and your meal is one hour or more away, or if your blood-sugar level drops and you fall into an energy slump. Always check in with yourself to see if you may be dehydrated instead of actually being hungry or if what you're experiencing is more a habit of distraction than the need for food.

Daily mealtimes

Breakfast is the most important meal of the day— you've probably heard it many times, and it's true! The best time to eat your breakfast is between 7 and 9 am, when your digestive system is the strongest. Breakfast is essential when you're starting your day since it helps to stabilize your blood-sugar levels after the night of fasting. It establishes a good consistent energy level for the day, helps you feel satisfied all morning, and keeps you from feeling hungry until lunch—at least if you choose a hearty, fiber-rich breakfast.

Some people feel they aren't hungry for breakfast in the morning. This is often a sign that their evening meal on the previous day was too big, too heavy, or eaten too late—which can easily be the case if you didn't eat regular meals throughout the day and then overate at night to compensate. Your body is simply unable to process and digest all that extra food overnight, and evening is also not when you need the energy. Daytime is! Remember, food is energy, which is really what calories mean: available energy.

It's a good idea to start getting used to eating breakfast. Studies have shown that mastering your weight is much easier when you eat breakfast, partly because it helps you feel more nourished as your day is getting going, and that helps you have better eating habits throughout the day.

Lunch is a meal that many people tend to keep small, eat fast, or skip altogether. But it's an important meal, providing a break in the middle of the day and an opportunity to recharge our batteries and refill our energy supply for the afternoon. When we don't eat lunch, we often end up feeling depleted by evening and we can overeat at dinner.

I also often see clients eating too light of a meal at lunch and then wondering why they're hungry again by 3pm, or why they feel tired and unable to concentrate in the afternoon. It's no accident that afternoon is the time when most people aren't able to master their cravings for something sweet and end up digging into the cookie jar or going to the vending machine. We've already learned that there's nothing wrong with a healthy snack when your next meal is one hour or more away, but these snack attacks that come after a too-light lunch tend to be of the unhealthy variety; it's just too difficult to master your cravings and make healthy choices when you are feeling depleted, and when your blood-sugar is low you can feel like you're starving.

The best way to keep your energy level steady and master your appetite throughout the day is to make breakfast and lunch the larger meals of your day. If you tend to need an afternoon snack, plan ahead for it and make sure you have healthy options on hand, like nuts or fresh fruit, carrots, hummus, or other small real-food items that you can carry with you. Trail mix can be a good portable option, but choose one higher in unsalted nuts and lower in fruit to avoid triggering the bliss-point. Soup is a great snack, too. Just remember: Think food first!

Dinner is—mistakenly—the main meal of the day for far too many people in our modern society. In fact, most of us tend to wait to eat the bulk of their food at dinnertime. If you have skimped on or skipped breakfast and lunch, or maybe just snacked all day, you are setting yourself up for overeating at night. You'll be depleted from exerting energy and not taking in any or enough fuel (food), and the end result is that at dinner, your body will try to refill the empty depot. It's like having pushed the car all day long only to get to the gas station in time to fuel up and leave it in the garage. Your appetite will be almost impossible to master because your body will interpret the lack of fuel as the threat of starvation—so it will trigger you to eat more than you need because your survival mechanism wants to pack away and hoard the food that's finally in front of you. It's not you; it is the nature of appetite, hunger, and satiation.

You'll feel much better overall if you can make this one change to your habits: Let dinner be the lighter meal of your day. You only need enough energy from dinner to last you until bedtime—which, as you've probably heard before, should fall at least two to three hours after you eat. This is because your body needs the night to restore, recover, and rebuild, not to work on digesting food. Eating too late causes bad sleep, acid reflux, and your body simply not getting enough rest and recovery overnight. Nighttime is also when the organs detox, which is one of the reasons you feel like a trainwreck in the morning if your dinner was excessive.

The idea of eating lighter at night is challenging for most people. This is the moment when we finally sit down to relax; with that, we tend to indulge. It's also the time we spend with family and friends. For many people, the evening meal is when we have the hardest time stopping and checking in with our satiety. When we feel lonely, tired, frustrated, stressed out—you name it—evening is when we're most liable to overeat or to go for sweet snacks, cookies, or ice cream. If this sounds familiar, it means that evening is when it's important for you to have a good plan for alternative activities that can make you feel nurtured and comforted, so food doesn't become your only choice.

TRICKS FOR MASTERING YOUR APPETITE AND CRAVINGS

- When eating, sit at the table and chew well; you'll feel more satisfied from less food if you do.

- Do not multi task, be on your phone or computer, or watch TV until the meal is over. You can plan to start a good film after the meal.

- Make sure your meal has a beginning and an end. A nice ritual may help you create these "bookends."

- Beware of under-eating at meals; it can easily lead to over-snacking later.

- To avoid overeating, serve only one portion on the plate, put the rest away for another meal or a snack-meal, so you avoid going for seconds.

- Drink water or tea after the meal so you allow some time to get a sense of your satiety level. Remember the twenty-minute rule.

- Remember: Food is energy!

MINDFUL EATING

Many of us, especially in a stressed environment, don't eat when we are hungry. Instead we eat when there is an opportunity to—or else we don't eat at all and ignore the hunger, we snack all day instead of eating a real meal, and/or we wait to get home at night and then indulge and overeat. Does any of this sound familiar? Maybe you've noticed that you're gaining pounds that seem to just sneak up on you—all of a sudden, you're ten pounds heavier than you were last year, and you didn't even notice it happening. There's an explanation for this: an extra 100 calories per day adds up to 10 pounds of weight gain per year. But 100 calories doesn't seem like a lot when you're eating it, does it?

It's a real challenge to keep in touch with our true appetites when we are under stress. It takes mindfulness not to grab that afternoon cookie or candy bar when we need to calm down a bit, or when we're tired and looking for some quick energy. You'll notice this especially on days when you've skipped lunch. It's very important to be aware of your snacking habits when you're trying to lose weight. Snacking is one of those habits that can easily become completely mindless, especially when we're stressed; this kind of snacking has nothing to do with hunger, it's just a way of temporarily calming us down.

THE GREAT BIG FOOD TRAPS

Study after study show how the human mind gets tricked by labels, words, enticing descriptions, and advertising. If left to its own devices, the unconscious mind will believe what it sees and hears, and we will eat whatever is labeled "healthy" without further scruples. So it seems that we cannot quite trust ourselves when making choices, unless we are mindfully participating in those choices. In other words; we have to actively use our mind to make conscious choices that support us in our health goals. This is a crucial aspect of getting healthy and changing eating habits. The unconscious mind won't be able to do so on its own. It needs you and your conscious mind to participate.

Here are a few culprits that have you adding extra mindless calories:

Time spent eating
Studies have shown that the average lunch meal in

a fast food restaurant takes 11 minutes, in a workplace cafeteria 13 minutes, and at a moderately priced restaurant 28 minutes. Take a moment right now to think back over your day:

- How much time do you allow for eating?

- Do you take a lunch break or do you rush some food in while doing something else?

- How much time do you spend at the table at dinner or for breakfast?

Your morning routine—including breakfast—can be harnessed to set up your unconscious mind to make the right choices for the day. If you give yourself a little more time in the morning to actually sit down for a bowl of hot breakfast cereal, for example, you are sending yourself a message that is very different than if you run out the door with a breakfast bar in hand or grab a bagel on the run. This choice will affect your eating habits for the rest of the day. Finding a routine in the morning that sets up a good rhythm for the day makes a huge difference in how you feel and how you take care of yourself.

Serving sizes

The size of a dish you are served in a restaurant or for take-out is often what you will end up eating. It's a function of how we eat when we eat mindlessly, but also of how many of us were brought up—to be members of the empty-plate club. Instead, consider the serving size you really want to eat when it arrives in front of you. Don't expect of yourself that you can stop eating in the middle of the meal—it's not fair to ask that of yourself, especially when you're just starting out with mindful eating. Put what you decide you don't need to the side, or ask for a separate plate put in onto. I know it will possibly feel a bit strange at first, but you can even ask for a "doggy bag" before you've started eating. Many of us are triggered by the feeling of having to finish what's on the plate instead of throwing it out. So don't throw it out—if you're in a city where there are homeless people on the street, you can give the food away before you even get home; otherwise, you can keep it for others in your household or for a meal for yourself the following day.

As you'll see in the section about reading labels, serving sizes can be deceiving. When a given amount of food lands our plate, we have to make a very conscious choice to leave some food behind if we want to avoid overeating. Mastering your appetite involves the mindful practice of learning to recognize when you have just started to feel full. If you can take a pause then, you're much less likely to pick up the fork again and overeat. The best thing is to move the plate away. If you're like me, picking at the food after eating can feel comforting, but it also adds another serving if you aren't mindful. Some say the best practice is to stop eating at the point when you are no longer feeling actively hungry, which can be really hard—so your best option is to learn to serve yourself smaller portions, knowing that if you are truly still hungry there is more food available. If you can find a way to pause before you feel full, then, twenty minutes later, you'll feel nicely satisfied instead of stuffed.

I don't want to pretend that this is easy. If you are used to feeling stuffed then it will feel "unsafe" to eat less, so take a gentle, steady, mindful, and kind approach towards yourself as you learn to sit with the emotions that are triggered when you feel anything less than over-full. Remember that our inherited survival instincts trigger our hunger, which is why you want to learn how to master your eating habits. Even though we may intellectually know that we can find food, as human beings we still have the instinct to avoid starvation however we can. If you can stay aware of the origins of this instinct, you'll be less likely to judge yourself for it. Also, for many of us, feeling stuffed is a safety zone for emotional reasons, not just our survival instincts; but this doesn't mean it's a true comfort zone. Mindfulness and self-compassion will help you recognize the difference.

Serving size illusions

We tend to decide in advance if a meal is going to satisfy us or not. When a little food is on a big plate, your mind gets triggered to think you're getting less food than if the same amount of food were on a smaller plate. This means that if you use smaller plates, your mind will think you're eating more than you are. Looking at a plate that's overflowing with food sends a message that you're about to eat a lot. This trick helps you unconsciously check in with your hunger and appetite much earlier in the meal—before you go for the next serving of food— and you'll have a chance to stop before overeating.

Too many choices

Variety makes us eat more. The buffet table and the salad bar can be traps for overeating. There is so much to taste, and you keep doing so. There's nothing wrong with tasting—as we've learned, variety is important. The problem is that in these all-you-can-eat situations, your mind gets triggered to enter survival mode: "Food is here. Eat while you can!" Also, every time you add a new and different taste, your appetite somehow gets re-activated; again, this is part of your survival mechanism, the very same one that has you devouring dessert even when you are already stuffed. So, learn to balance variety with simplicity so you'll be able to know when you're fully satiated.

See food, eat food

When you see it, you want it. It's human nature to want to eat "everything in sight." This means that if you aren't mindful, you'll probably reach for that cookie even if you're not really hungry. To master your appetite, cravings, and eating habits, stay mindful and keep easy-to-grab foods and snacks out of sight. Because once you start dipping into the office cookie stash or the bowl of chocolates on your desk, it's that much harder to stop.

Who, me?

Who is eating? When you are on email, watching TV, or driving, you are not mindful of the fact you're eating, let alone how much you're eating, since your mind is elsewhere. So stick to one thing at a time. Have you noticed how sometimes your plate is empty and suddenly you realize you have no clue what the food tasted like or where it went? It's as if your mind was eating something entirely different from the food on your plate. When this happens, since you've missed out on all of the pleasurable aspects of eating, you'll instinctively want to eat "again" (or more)—while paying attention this time. (Even though it's likely you'll be just as unfocused the second time around!) This is what happens with mindless eating—we end up feeling as if we are not even there. To master your appetite, make sure your mind is focused on your food when you eat. It's an active effort!

The trouble with the label "Healthy Choice'

When "Healthy Choice" or similar claims are made on a label, it doesn't always mean that the food is actually healthy. It can mean that the calories are healthier ones—which is good—but there still might be the same number of calories as in an unhealthy food. You need to be mindful of how *much* you eat, even when it's healthy—and don't get fooled into mindless eating by names and words that are designed to sell you a product. Many think that when a food is labeled healthy its calories don't "count" and you can eat more. It's up to you to practice mindful choices and to be a full participant in determining what's healthy for you. Taking responsibility for the choices you make about what you eat might feel like a chore at first, but after a little practice you will feel so much more empowered, because you KNOW.

Sounds yummy

Your brain decides in advance if you're going to find a food delicious. So if it sounds great on the menu, you're more likely to eat it all up. It's important to love the taste of your food—I believe this is essential to eating well and feeling good. But you don't want a marketing description to decide what's delicious: it's better to leave that up to your taste-buds and your body. Also, when we assume something is going to be really yummy we tend to eat it too fast. Instead, slow down and enjoy it even more—you're allowed! Then you can really eat with pleasure and master your appetite and your cravings at the same time.

→ Remember that our inherited survival instincts trigger our hunger.

→ Mindfulness and self-compassion can help us know when we are truly hungry and when we are seeking another kind of comfort.

→ The buffet table and the salad bar can be traps for overeating. Learn to balance variety with simplicity.

→ Try using smaller plates to trick your mind into thinking you're eating more than you are.

→ Let your mind be focused on your food when you eat. Eating is an activity!

EATING MORE OR LESS

Choice

According to research, the average person makes more than 200 food choices per day. Do you realize how many times a day that means you have food on your mind? Granted, for many of us these are mostly unconscious thoughts and choices that we aren't aware of. But if you struggle with food, it can seem as if it's the only thing on your mind.

The questions are many: what to eat, how, when, where, how much, and so on. We are often obsessed with food because we're triggered by the smells and sight of it everywhere. It follows us at every step, in our daily conversations, TV ads, cooking shows, and more. So that's why the question to ask yourself is: Am I making conscious choices or absent-minded choices, and are these choices what I want or are they the result of sheer habit? I had a client who was working really hard on mastering her appetite, but she was finding it impossible not to snack at night. Then we finally realized that she was in the habit of watching cooking shows after dinner, and seeing all that food on the screen was what was sending her back to the cupboard for more!

The unconscious mind and the hidden ways of persuasion are very interesting and sometimes quite scary. In one study, a single nanosecond-long glimpse of a beverage was added into a movie strip. This was too fast for the conscious mind to pick up, but not so for the unconscious mind. As a result of it, viewers bought more soda at intermission and even left the theater in the midst of the movie to get a refill.

Size

We tend to eat more of a packaged food that is packaged in a larger size. It's like a subconscious message that tells us whatever size the package is must be the appropriate serving size. Too often we forget not only to check in with our stomachs to see if we actually want the whole thing, but also to read the label and see if the package contains more than one serving. In addition, serving sizes are hard to understand because they're actually just a measure of units that makes it possible to compare products—they don't always correspond to the serving you're meant to eat. And then of course each of us is different, and we need different portion sizes.

In a nutshell: A serving size is not always your portion size. A package is not always your portion either.

Serving sizes have grown over the years. Today, the size of movie-theater soda is anything from 2–4 servings, so that a person can order—and drink!—a 32-ounce bucket of the stuff. The official size for one serving of soda is 8 ounces, and in this case I suggest that to be your maximum portion size as well.

Calories are listed on all packaged foods, but so are percentages of Daily Nutritional Values. Many Americans consume more calories than they need without actually meeting the recommended intake for nutrients. While I don't recommend trying to get your nutrients from real ingredients in packaged foods, always check labels to make sure that at least you aren't consuming a lot of empty calories. If the calorie count is high and all or most of the nutrient percentages are low or added artificially, there's not much value to the food and it's better to avoid it altogether. This is what is meant by *wasting calories*.

Understanding quality versus quantity

There are several very important things to look for on labels. Look for the word "whole," such as wholegrain wheat instead of just whole wheat, which is really only slightly less refined than white flour. Foods marked with words such as "multigrain," "stone-ground," "100% wheat," "cracked wheat," "seven-grain," or "bran" are not necessarily wholegrain products. Color is also not an indication of a food being wholegrain. Brown and darker bread isn't necessarily made from wholegrain flours. Some brown bread has caramel color added to give it a brown tone, making us think we're buying something healthy—it can all be very confusing. There is an official stamp you can look for, the "Wholegrain "stamp. It will indicate either "good source," which contains at least a half-serving of wholegrain or "excellent source," which contains at least one full serving of wholegrain. Still, cooked wholegrain dishes are better than flour products, even if they are made from wholegrain flour.

→ Ask yourself: Am I making conscious choices about what and how often I eat, or am I acting out of habit?

→ Know the difference between serving size, portion size, and package size.

READING LABELS

It's essential to read all the ingredients on the label. The first ingredient listed on a packaged food is what there is most of, and the amount of each ingredient decreases from there. Make sure that the first several ingredients on a label are real food, not sugar or chemical additives! But read all of the ingredients so you can be sure that no non-food substances have been added—usually these appear toward the bottom of the list, since they are often used in small quantities (which doesn't make them healthy). A good rule of thumb is: If you can't tell from the name of an ingredient what kind of whole food it came from, it's not worth eating. You also need to read the fine print below the label, where all the little extras sneak in that have lower values than what need to be specified by labeling laws.

Currently it's not a national requirement to label GMO ingredients, but there is a big push to make this happen. Until it does, be extra careful of any packaged foods that contain corn and soy, since in commercial products these ingredients are almost always from genetically modified sources. More and more, you'll see that companies are producing packaged foods labeled GMO-free; this fortunately takes some of the guesswork out of it until the labeling laws change to give us the full picture of what's in our foods.

One of the most important values to look for is the sugar content and source. Look for the word "sugar" or even "brown sugar" and note how far up it's listed. If it's one of the first ingredients, then you know that you're eating mostly sugar! Also, be aware of other names for sugar, such as fruit juice concentrate, and do try to completely avoid foods with corn syrup and high-fructose corn syrup; also limit those containing maltose, dextrose, and sucrose. It is also best to stay away from the artificial sweeteners such as saccharin, aspartame, acesulfame potassium, sucralose, neotame, and cyclamate. These are all on the warning list for cancer. There are sugar substitutes from common brand-names that use these ingredients, so just because you don't see the brand name here, still check the ingredients, since these are still best avoided.

Better sources of sweetener to look for are the more natural and less-processed options, such as raw cane sugar, brown rice syrup, honey, maple syrup, molasses, agave nectar, and stevia (even though this is referred to as an artificial sweetener, it is actually a natural product derived from a leaf—however, it is highly processed). Foods sweetened with fruit or raw cane sugar are better than those sweetened with refined sugar, but all sweetened foods have high glycemic indexes and you'll still want to consume them in moderation, if at all.

Another trick about reading labels for sugar content: Carbohydrates are listed as total carbohydrates; below that, sugars are listed separately. (There is some indication that food labels will be changing in the future.) In foods that contain sugar, look for it to be balanced by fiber; the presence of fiber in foods that contain sugar lowers their glycemic index and will result in steadier insulin levels. We've already learned how important insulin levels are to health and to the mastering of our appetites.

The next value to look for is the fat content, as well as the source of the fats. Is it saturated (from an animal source and best limited) or is it unsaturated (from a vegetable source and a better choice)? If a product says it's fat-free, don't buy it. As you have already learned, this often means you will have no or little satisfaction from this food, plus the sugar content is typically very high in fat-free packaged foods.

The fiber content is crucial for mastering your appetite but also for your health. As I keep repeating (and for good reason), we always want to get as much fiber from our food as possible. This is what helps us on our path to more health, a feeling of satiety, and more sustainable energy.

Just to remind you, high fiber content slows down the absorption time of glucose and extends its available distribution. This means both longer lasting energy and the feeling of being full for a longer period.

Again, the greatest confusion is that all the values listed on a label are calculated per serving, and a serving size is not necessarily the same as what goes on your plate—or even what's recommended. For example, for a balanced meal you want to have one portion size of protein, which is 4-6 oz. (like fish or legumes or meat), but 3–5 servings of vegetables, which is several cups of veggies.

What is important is the quality of the food you are choosing because that becomes the quality of how you feel.

→ If you can't tell from the name of an ingredient what kind of whole food it came from, it's not worth eating.

→ If a product says it's fat-free, don't buy it.

→ The quality of your food translates into the quality of your sense of well-being.

THE SELF-NOURISHMENT ~~DIET~~

The simple outline of eating for self-nourishment is:

- Cooked grain with nuts and seeds, optional egg, and even vegetables in the morning

- Legumes or other vegan protein sources with high-fiber vegetables (roots, cruciferous, and leafy greens) for lunch.

- Fish and greens for dinner (unless you're vegan—then you can get your protein from legumes, tempeh, or quinoa).

The thing to remember is that how you eat does not have to have a name, it just has to be nourishing for you!

THE FOOD-MIND-BODY CONNECTION

Now that you have read this book, take a moment to settle into your body in a comfortable chair. Notice how you feel in your body. It's such a nice practice to notice how you feel in your body. Read the following first, or have someone read it to you. Then close your eyes.

Visualize YOU being active and moving around feeling vibrant and healthy. Get a sense that you have finished the day of work or are taking a break to eat, and you're looking forward to a good meal. Now imagine yourself sitting down at the table, looking at a plate that's rich with fresh vegetables and foods that nourish you. Take a nice deep breath, and just have simple gratitude for the food and all it has gone through to get to you. Include all the people who have been involved in growing it, transporting it, selling it, and cooking it (especially if that is you). Before you start to eat, enjoy the sight of your food while knowing that it will nourish you, satisfy you, and keep you content and satiated for hours to come.

Take one more nice nourishing breath, and make note of how you now feel in your body when I say "food."

Enjoy eating, savor every bite, and know that you are taking good care of your Self in the process. That is what self-nourishment is: *you* taking really good care of *you*, eating foods that nourish and nurture the whole of *you*. Your body, your mind, and your soul. Eat with all your senses, and you will feel so much more nourished.

"I make a big pot of brown rice or wholegrain because it keeps for several days in the fridge."

COOKING BASICS

These recipes offer basic guidelines for cooking ingredients in the food groups you've learned about in this book. You can freely mix them together for a nourishing meal, adding spices and herbs to taste, and adjusting portions to serve a friend or a group or just to make a nourishing meal for yourself.

I invite you to play with cooking—have fun, and find the most satisfying way for *you* to eat to feel full.

Brown Rice / Ancient Grains
The simplest and easiest way to add some good substance to a meal.

Ingredients (per person)
Brown rice or any wholegrain - 1/2 cup
Water - 1 1/2 cup
Pinch of sea salt

Method
Cooking time is 45-55 min. on a simmer.

Rinse rice or other wholegrain three times in a colander. Bring the rice/grain and water to a boil, then lower the heat to a simmer. Leave the lid slightly ajar so the steam can escape. Start checking it at 35 min. When it's almost cooked with just a little water on top, turn off the heat and let it sit for another 15 min. Don't ever stir your rice/grain. You can, of course, cook most wholegrain in a rice cooker, which offers the benefit of automatically shutting off when the grain is perfectly cooked— but the above method is just as foolproof once you've gotten the hang of it. You will need to remember to set your timer, though!

Optional: Pre-soak your grain.
When you soak rice or grain overnight before cooking it, the starch content will be lower and the grain will cook faster. Soak in plenty of water overnight, then rinse at least once in fresh water. Discard the rinse water and add fresh water before cooking. The instructions are otherwise the same, but you'll want to check the grain at about 25 minutes because of the faster cooking time.

I tend to make a big pot of rice or whole grain (my favorites are brown rice, whole oats, barley, and sometimes sweet brown rice) because it keeps for several days in the fridge. That way breakfast is easy, and any mix of grain salads is always a fast option. You can use a regular pot—stainless steel, clay, or enamel—and leave the lid slightly ajar, but I prefer to use a donabe pot: These clay pots have rounded bottoms, which are ideal for cooking rice and grain, and they have a steam hole in the lid to ensure the grain does not boil over.

If you want to cook for more days or more people, follow these rules of thumb: 1 cup of rice or other whole-grain needs 2 1/2 cups of water. Cook with a pinch of salt. 1 cup uncooked rice or whole-grain makes 2 cups cooked.

Cooked Root Vegetables

Roasting (or baking) roots requires some up-front labor, but once the vegetables are chopped, it's easy! And oven-cooked roots go so well with many dishes. Basically, you can choose any root you like; they all cook the same way.

Ingredients
Sweet potatoes
Parsnip or turnip (or both)
Carrots
Onion

Sea salt
Herbs

Method
Preheat the oven to 425 degrees. Peel and cube roots into bite-size pieces (or smaller, if you want a sort of chunky hash). Put them in a baking dish, and pour a little oil over them (you can also use water or tea). Add spices if you like; I often use fresh-ground coriander seed and whole pepper corn. Check and stir after about 25-30 min. You'll need to add a little water to the bottom of the pan to make sure the roots don't dry out too much. The roots should take about 45 minutes to be roasted to perfection.

Roasted Cauliflower
Roasting cauliflower makes it nice and crispy, and you can add different herbs and spices for different flavors, which makes it rather versatile as well.

Ingredients
Cauliflower
Untoasted sesame oil or other high-heat oil
Sea salt
Herbs

Method
Preheat the oven to 425 degrees. Cut the stems of the cauliflower to leave the "flower" parts whole. Spread the cut cauliflower in a baking dish and add a little cooking oil appropriate for high-heat cooking—I like untoasted sesame oil. Add some sea salt, pepper, and herbs to your liking: sage, curry, herbes de Provence, rosemary—really anything will work. Cook for about 35 minutes. You might want to stir and toss a couple of times, but otherwise it pretty much takes care of itself. Serve with a grain dish, lentils or fish, and other good veggies, of course!

Sautéed Red Cabbage

Sautéing is one of the easiest methods for cooking vegetables: Just cut them up, add them to a hot pan with a little oil, and stir gently with a wooden spoon. Cabbage is one of the foods that I only learned to like when I tasted it sautéed.

Ingredients
Cabbage
Sea salt
Untoasted sesame oil
Mirin

Method

Chop the cabbage into strips. Heat a sauté pan over medium heat. Add a little oil, a dash of salt, and the cabbage. Stir the cabbage gently with a wooden spoon. It will probably need more liquid—you can use more oil, but I tend to use a little mirin to let the sweetness of the cabbage come through. You can also add some tea if you have pot of it sitting around. Cabbage needs a bit more time than leafy greens. It's up to you how crunchy you prefer it, but look for the color to turn. Once it's bright, it's ready. If you want it softer, you can keep going—the more you cook it, the sweeter it gets.

Sautéed Greens

Sautéing greens is a fast and easy way to a healthy meal.

Ingredients
Collard greens, or any other dark leafy greens
Garlic
Sea salt
Untoasted sesame oil

Method
Cut the collard greens into strips. If you choose another dark leafy green, you can either chop it or

cut into strips. Peel the garlic; you can leave the cloves whole or cut them in half. Start them up on low to medium heat with the oil. When they are turning slightly brown—about 10-15 minutes—add the greens and stir together. The greens only need a few minutes on the heat; when they turn bright green, they're ready.

Sautéed Onions & Leeks

Onions and leeks are a great addition to many meals but are also fantastic on their own, as a side-dish. Or cook up a portion and keep them on hand to mix into other meals.

Ingredients
Onion(s)
Leek(s)
Untoasted sesame oil

Method
You can use this method to cook a mixture of onions and leeks in any proportion, or cook just one or the other. For onions, peel and cut into thick whole or half rings; for leeks, cut off the ends, take the outer layer off, and slice into rings. Add oil and the onion and leek to the pan, and sauté over medium heat. (When you heat up cooking oil at the same time as

onions, their sweetness comes out more.) As the pan starts to dry up, add a dash of sea salt, which will draw some of the moisture out of the onions and leeks. Keep stirring, and if you need to you can add a little water. You can also use tea, or mirin, or another cooking vinegar that is not too acidic, like brown rice vinegar or apple cider vinegar. If you want a crispier texture, add only a few drops of liquid; for a softer consistency and sweeter taste, you can add a little more.

Marinated Kale Salad

My favorite easy-to-make kale salad that goes with everything.

Ingredients

Kale (curly kale is best)

Sea salt

Olive oil

Mirin, brown rice vinegar, or lemon juice

Method

Chop the kale finely. You can make the whole bunch at once, or just enough for one meal (at least 5 stems of kale). I normally make the whole bunch at a time because it holds up so well in the fridge. Put all the chopped kale in a stainless steel or glass bowl, drizzle a large dash of sea salt over it (about

1–2 teaspoons, depending on how much kale you are making), and start massaging with your hands. Add some mirin, brown-rice vinegar, or lemon juice. Keep massaging, then add the olive oil.

Find a plate that's smaller than the diameter of your bowl. Place the plate directly on top of the kale and press it down. You might want to put a rock or something heavy on top of the plate to add pressure. Let the kale be pressed for a good 20 minutes before serving. (You can omit this step if you have massaged it really well.) You can keep marinated kale in the fridge for a at least another day.

Lentil Salad
Lentils cook really fast and can be used on their own as a salad or as part of a dish. They're an excellent source of protein, but they also add some substance to a lighter meal.

Ingredients (per person)
1/2 cup of dry lentils (1 cup dry makes 1 cup cooked lentils—a full portion, good enough for a meal. If you're using the lentils as part of a meal, you might just want about 1/2 -3/4 cup cooked of lentils per person)

Water (1 1/4 cups per 1/2 cup of lentils)
Sea salt and pepper to taste

Method
Wash the lentils in a colander and add to a pot with the water. Wait to add salt and pepper until the lentils are cooked. You can add herbs if you like while cooking. Bring to a boil, then lower to a simmer. Cook with the lid ajar for 20-25 min. Check periodically to make sure the lentils aren't getting dry. You can add a little water if they are too al dente; it depends on how you like them. When cooked, add sea salt and pepper to taste. To serve, mix with anything chopped. You can mix in kale or any other greens, peas, string beans, broccoli, cauliflower, carrots, sweet potato—anything goes, really. If you have leftovers, this is a great way to put together a salad. If you want to cook the vegetables in with the lentils, you can do that too. Roots take about the same time to boil so that works well; if you want to add in a green vegetable, just put them into the pot for the last 5 minutes of cooking time only. Mix with olive oil, serve and enjoy.

Cooked Beans

The recipe below is for fava beans, but any bean can be used: white beans, canellini beans, red beans, black beans, adzuki beans. Cook them in advance to be mixed in with a variety of dishes, or serve them as a side dish.

Ingredients
Fava beans or other bean, dry (about 1/2 cup per person)
Garlic (optional)

Method
For cooking dry beans, soak overnight, rinse in a colander and use either a pressure cooker or a pot to cook.

Pressure Cooker: Avoid putting herbs in with the beans, as they can clog the steam holes. It took me a while to get used to using a pressure cooker because I was afraid of all the stories about the thing flying through the air under too much pressure. Well, it seems those stories might be outdated. Pressure cookers save time, taking about 25-45 minutes to cook beans (compared to 90 minutes or more in a pot on the stove). I tend to add a whole dry shiitake mushroom to add flavor—but no salt (that goes in afterwards). Garlic and kombu are optional, but help with the digestion of beans. After pressure-cooking, add sea salt to taste, along with any other herbs, and leave on the stove top to cook for another 5 min.

Stove top: When cooking beans in a pot, you can add the garlic and herbs at the start, but still leave out the sea salt until the beans are done. Different beans have different cooking times, so you might want to look these up, but you can estimate at least 90 minutes for most beans on the stove top.

Tempeh

Cooking tempeh can seem like a big effort at first, but it is really fast once you get the hang of it.

Ingredients
Tempeh
Untoasted sesame oil
Mirin
Tamari (gluten free)

Method
Preheat oven to 425 degrees. Cut the tempeh into cubes—you can make them thicker or thinner depending on what you like. I like my tempeh cooked really well so it gets crispy. First I braise it on the stove top for about 10 minutes (5 on each side) and then I put it in the oven to bake for 20-30 minutes.

In the pan, I add about a tablespoon of oil and a dash of mirin and tamari soy sauce. This is optional, but I like the taste of the glaze that results. You will need to add a little water because the tempeh soaks up a lot of liquid—which is why I use water instead of extra oil. A cast iron pan is best for this. After the sauté, put it in the oven with a little water in the bottom of the pan. You can turn the tempeh over once or twice while it's in the oven. I add a little more water along the way when it seems to get dry. Let it bake for about 20-30 minutes depending on how crispy you like it. The herbs and spices I like with this dish are crushed whole peppercorn (1 teaspoon), a little sea salt (large dash), and a medium dash (1/2 teaspoon) of cayenne. How much you use is up to your taste buds. Try it yourself!

Whole Roasted Fish

Roasting a whole fish is rather easy and makes for a great presentation.

Ingredients
Choice of whole fish
Any fresh herb

Method
Preheat oven to 425 degrees. Rinse the fish and

stuff with herbs. You can add some sea salt and freshly ground pepper to both the inside and out-side of the fish. Put a little oil in the bottom of a baking dish, then add the fish. Bake uncovered for 15-20 minutes, depending on the size and stuffing (a fish with more stuffing will require a little more time). Check for doneness with a sharp knife—if you feel resistance, leave it in a bit longer. Serve with sautéed greens, roots, vegetables—anything goes well with a whole fish.

Fish & Greens

This dish of marinated kale and a baked fillet of fish is deeply satisfying and easy to digest. When eaten as an evening meal, it gives your body a good rest overnight.

Ingredients
1 fillet of white fish (per person)
Untoasted sesame oil
Marinated kale
Sea salt, pepper, herbs

Method
Preheat oven to 425 degrees. Add a little cooking oil to a baking dish, then add the fillet and sprinkle

with sea salt, freshly ground pepper, and/or herbs to your liking. Bake uncovered for 12-15 minutes, depending on how cooked through you want it. Plate with marinated kale (see recipe above), and enjoy!

Spending time with your Self while eating is a nourishing way to pause and care for YOU.

"The meals I cook for myself are ingredient driven. That allows me to be creative with what I have in the fridge."

SHOPPING LIST

VEGETABLES
Cruciferous Family
Broccoli, Broccoli Rabe, Bok Choy, Brussels Sprouts, Cabbage, Cauliflower, Collards, Kale

Allium Family
Onion, Leeks, Scallions

Leafy & Other Greens
Asparagus, Artichokes, String Beans, Peas, Arugula, Mesclun, Watercress, Spinach* (avoid if inflammation, acid reflux, arthritis, osteoporosis, or anemia are issues)

* Spinach belongs to the nightshade family, vegetables that are best consumed only in small amounts. Other nightshade vegetables are: Tomatoes, Peppers, Egglpant, Zucchini, White Potatoes. Tobacco and coffee are also nightshades.

Roots, Tubers, & Winter Squash
Carrots, Beets, Parsnips, Turnips, Sweet Potatoes, Yams, Winter Squash (Butternut, Acorn, & Pumpkin)

Mushrooms
Shiitake, Maitake, Morel, Porcini, Oyster, Portobello, Dried Wild Mushrooms (to be reconstituted with water)

Wholegrain
Gluten-free choices: Brown, Red, Black & Wild Rice, Millet, Quinoa, Oats (choose gluten free), Buckwheat, Amaranth, Teff, Corn*

Choices that contain gluten: Kamut, Spelt, Rye, Barley, Couscous*, Wheat*

PLANT PROTEIN
Legumes
Beans, Lentils, Peas, Chickpeas, Hummus

Nuts
Walnuts, Pecans, Almonds, Pistachios, Pine Nuts, Cashews, Brazil Nuts

Seeds
Pumpkin Seeds, Sunflower Seeds, Sesame Seeds, Chia Seeds, Hemp Seeds, Flax Seeds

Nut Butters
Butters made from nuts and seeds (only without added sugar or hydrogenated oil)

Soy Products*
Tempeh, Cooked Tofu, Edamame*, Miso

Other
Quinoa, Avocado

ANIMAL PROTEIN
Fish
Fresh Small and White Fish (Cod, Halibut, Flounder, Sole, etc.), Wild Salmon, Swordfish**, Tuna**

Meat
Only Organic Grass Fed and Free Range Lamb & Beef, Wild Game

* Always choose non-GMO
** Max 1x Weekly

Poultry & Eggs
Organic and Free-Range Eggs, Chicken, Turkey

"Milks"
Rice Milk, Almond Milk, Hemp Milk, Oat Milk,
Coconut Milk

Note: Most adults are lactose intolerant—and
we are supposed to be by nature—so avoid cow's
milk. Avoid soy milk.

FATS
For cooking: Untoasted Sesame Oil, Coconut Oil,
Olive Oil, Nut and Avocado Oil

To add after cooking: Virgin Cold Expelled Olive
Oil, Flax Oil, Hemp Oil, Sesame and Nut Oils

SWEETENERS
Use only natural sweeteners.
Raw Honey, Real Maple Syrup, Brown Rice Syrup,
Real Cane Sugar, Agave Nectar, (Stevia)

LIQUIDS

Spring or Filtered Water, Herbal Teas, White Tea, Green Tea, Oolong Tea, Pu-erh Tea, Black Tea (occasionally), Green & Vegetable Juices (wheat grass, spirulina, leafy greens), Vegetable Juices (leafy greens, carrot, beet, celery, cucumber. Add apple, lemon, or ginger for taste.)

ANTI-INFLAMMATORY CONDIMENTS

Cinnamon, Cumin, Garlic, Ginger, Rosemary, Turmeric

BEST AVOIDED

For healthy shopping and eating, it's best to avoid buying these foods.

Refined Sugar, Processed Food, Baked Goods, Cakes, Cookies, Refined Flour, Bread & Pasta, Potato Chips and other Salty Snack Foods, Candy, Gum, Soda, Food Coloring, Artificial Sweeteners, Preservatives

EAT TO FEEL FULL

Factory-Farm Raised Meats and Poultry, Eggs &
Dairy Products Packaged Meats, Bacon, Cold-
Cuts, Hot Dogs, Sausages

Fried Foods, Canned and Packaged Meals,
Non-Organic Coffee, Tea and Chocolate, Excess
Alcohol (no more than 2-3 drinks per week),
GMO-Foods & Non-Organic Foods in general

"We are always in a process of becoming. The more consciously you follow your Path, the more growth you will experience along the way."

AFTERWORD

Thank you for reading this book. When things end, something new begins. This is your new beginning, and I hope your journey will be tasty, nourishing, curious, and truly full of continuous wellness, happiness, and discovery of your Self. And—of course—full of satisfying, nourishing meals.

My own journey has gone on for many years. I don't know that I can even remember when it started. I do know that I have been and always will be on a Path—I don't know where or when it will end, but I enjoy the journey. It keeps surprising me, teaching me. I keep growing.

Everyone we meet is a teacher. Everything is a relationship. Everything is interaction. Every struggle we face teaches us something about ourselves. Every mistake we make is a step towards success, even when it can feel like failure in the moment. We can learn to cherish the precious moments, to invoke more joy and nourishment in everything we experience—and we can even learn to embrace the challenges. We are always in a process of becoming, and the more consciously you follow your Path, the more growth you will experience along the way.

I created my online program, Path for Life Self-Nourishment, to provide guidance to others who are seeking their own Path toward self-nourishment. Each of the nine steps is built around learning in three essential areas: food-knowledge, mindfulness, and habit-shifting. Together, they are designed to help you truly begin again, by creating a new relationship with food.

When I decided to devote myself to the practice and teaching of self-nourishment, I was in a moment of transition. I had left the fashion business, my own design firm, and a steadily growing career and income. My parents had both died from cancer one year apart from each other, and I found myself looking for answers and for a new life that I could call my own.

I found the answers within myself. And I keep finding them within myself. I hope you will too, and that with this book and with those that follow it, I can be your guide.

ACKNOWLEDGMENTS

Thank you to my husband, Torkil, for always being there to cheer me on, cook with me, and create amazing photographs that help make everyone want to cook and eat great food. Thank you to my clients who keep inspiring me to look deeper and further for what it takes to learn, grow, and change. Thank you to my tireless editor Anna, who keeps figuring out how to best translate what I'm trying to say. Thank you to all my teachers along the way, and most of all to Tom Monte, whom I met at a time when I decided to follow my passion even though I didn't know if my new lifestyle and career would make any sense. What I wanted was simple: to help people find joy. As a child with a chronically depressed parent, my greatest wish was for people to be happy. I would look at people I met and study them to try to understand who they were, to the point that my mom had to apologize for my "behavior." That desire to understand others has become my work today—seeing who is "in there," longing to come out, be seen, heard, embraced. Self-nourishment is how we give ourselves that opportunity. When I was confused about who I was becoming, Tom Monte helped me find my way. Thank you, Tom, for being my guide.

Jeanette Bronée founded Path for Life in 2004 to bring awareness to the healing power of learning how our choices affect us. She developed the nine-step, on-line Path For Life Self-Nourishment Program based on her integrative, mind-body approach to nourishment. An AADP board-certified Integrative Nutrition Health Coach, she holds additional certifications as a Meta-Medicine Coach®, Focusing Oriented Professional and Trainer, Ericksonian Hypnotherapist, EFT practitioner, and Connective Healing and Intuitive Counselor (with Tom Monte) and has been trained in Macrobiotic Healing and Energy Psychology. When not working one-one-one with her clients to develop individualized programs for self-nourishment, she is a writer, recipe developer, and motivational speaker. For more information, visit jeanettebronee.com.

PATH FOR LIFE BOOKS